Therapeutic Interaction in Nursing

SECOND EDITION

Christine L. Williams, DNSc, APRN, BC

Professor, Christine E. Lynn College of Nursing
Florida Atlantic University
Boca Raton, Florida

JONES AND BARTLETT PUBLISHERS

Sudbury, Massachusetts

BOSTON   TORONTO   LONDON   SINGAPORE

World Headquarters
Jones and Bartlett Publishers
40 Tall Pine Drive
Sudbury, MA 01776
978-443-5000
info@jbpub.com
www.jbpub.com

Jones and Bartlett Publishers Canada
6339 Ormindale Way
Mississauga, Ontario L5V 1J2
Canada

Jones and Bartlett Publishers International
Barb House, Barb Mews
London W6 7PA
United Kingdom

Jones and Bartlett's books and products are available through most bookstores and online booksellers. To contact Jones and Bartlett Publishers directly, call 800-832-0034, fax 978-443-8000, or visit our website www.jbpub.com.

Substantial discounts on bulk quantities of Jones and Bartlett's publications are available to corporations, professional associations, and other qualified organizations. For details and specific discount information, contact the special sales department at Jones and Bartlett via the above contact information or send an email to specialsales@jbpub.com.

The authors, editor, and publisher have made every effort to provide accurate information. However, they are not responsible for errors, omissions, or for any outcomes related to the use of the contents of this book and take no responsibility for the use of the products and procedures described. Treatments and side effects described in this book may not be applicable to all people; likewise, some people may require a dose or experience a side effect that is not described herein. Drugs and medical devices are discussed that may have limited availability controlled by the Food and Drug Administration (FDA) for use only in a research study or clinical trial. Research, clinical practice, and government regulations often change the accepted standard in this field. When consideration is being given to use of any drug in the clinical setting, the health care provider or reader is responsible for determining FDA status of the drug, reading the package insert, and reviewing prescribing information for the most up-to-date recommendations on dose, precautions, and contraindications, and determining the appropriate usage for the product. This is especially important in the case of drugs that are new or seldom used.

Production Credits
Executive Editor: Kevin Sullivan
Acquisitions Editor: Emily Ekle
Associate Editor: Amy Sibley
Editorial Assistant: Patricia Donnelly
Production Director: Amy Rose
Associate Production Editor: Wendy Swanson
Senior Marketing Manager: Katrina Gosek
Associate Marketing Manager: Rebecca Wasley
Manufacturing and Inventory Coordinator: Amy Bacus
Text Design: Lyn Rodger, Deerfoot Studios
Composition: Lyn Rodger, Deerfoot Studios
Cover Design: Kristin E. Ohlin
Cover Image: © Corbis Collection/Alamy Images
Printing and Binding: Courier Stoughton
Cover Printing: Courier Stoughton

Library of Congress Cataloging-in-Publication Data
Williams, Christine L., 1943-
   Therapeutic interaction in nursing / Christine L. Williams. — 2nd ed.
      p. ; cm.
   Includes bibliographical references and index.
   ISBN-13: 978-0-7637-5129-6 (pbk. : alk. paper)
   ISBN-10: 0-7637-5129-4 (pbk. : alk. paper) 1. Nurse and patient. 2. Communication in nursing. 3. Interpersonal communication. 4. Nurses—Psychology. I. Title.
   [DNLM: 1. Nurse-Patient Relations. 2. Communication. 3. Nurses—psychology. WY 87 W722t 2008]
   RT86.W557 2008
   610.7306'99—dc22
                              2007020673

6048
Printed in the United States of America
11 10 09 08 07   10 9 8 7 6 5 4 3 2 1

DEDICATION

This book is dedicated to the memory of my daughter Lauren and

to my daughter Kimberlee who brings me joy every day.

Contents

About the Author — *vii*

Contributors — *viii*

Preface — *ix*

Acknowledgments — *x*

SECTION 1 — THERAPEUTIC USE OF SELF

1. Understanding Ourselves and Our Relationships — 3
   (Christine L. Williams and Carol M. Davis)

2. Using the Self to Promote Health — 17
   (Christine L. Williams and Carol M. Davis)

SECTION 2 — INTERACTING WITH OTHERS

3. The Process of Helping — 29
   (Christine L. Williams and Carol M. Davis)

4. Communication Strategies — 41
   (Christine L. Williams)

5. Cross-Cultural Communication — 51
   (Tamika R. Sanchez-Jones)

6. Communicating with Families — 59
   (Christine L. Williams and Tamika R. Sanchez-Jones)

SECTION 3 — COMMUNICATING IN SPECIAL CIRCUMSTANCES

7. Communicating with Children — 69
   (Lois S. Marshall)

8. Communicating with Older Adults — 79
   (Theris A. Touhy and Christine L. Williams)

9. Communicating with Cognitively Impaired Persons — 91
   (Christine L. Williams and Ruth M. Tappen)

10. Communicating with Critically Ill, Mechanically Ventilated Clients — 105
    (Nancy E. Villanueva)

11. Communicating with Clients Experiencing Psychiatric Illness — 111
    (Christine L. Williams)

12. Communicating with Laboring Women — 123
    (Diane J. Angelini)

13. Communicating at Times of Loss and Grief — 131
    (Christine L. Williams)

14. Health Literacy and Communication — 139
    (Jackie H. Jones and Tamika R. Sanchez-Jones)

Index — *147*

About the Author

CHRISTINE L. WILLIAMS, DNSc, APRN, BC received a baccalaureate degree in nursing from Fitchburg State College in Massachusetts, a master's degree in Advanced Psychiatric Nursing of Adults from Rutgers University, and a Doctor of Nursing Science degree from Boston University. She is Board Certified by the ANCC as a Clinical Specialist in Psychiatric Mental Health Nursing and Gerontological Nursing. Currently, she is Professor in the Christine E. Lynn College of Nursing, Florida Atlantic University, Boca Raton, Florida. Dr. Williams has extensive experience teaching at the undergraduate and graduate levels. She has completed a number of studies on communication, aging, cultural, and mental health issues. She has been the recipient of grants from the National Institute for Nursing Research and private foundations. Dr. Williams is the author of many articles on aging, mental health, and communication.

Contributors

Diane J. Angelini, EdD, CNM, FACNM, FAAN, CNAA, BC
Clinical Associate Professor
Warren Alpert Medical School of Brown University
Director, Nurse Midwifery
Women and Infants' Hospital
Providence, Rhode Island

Carol M. Davis, DPT, EdD, MS, FAPTA
Professor and Assistant Chair
Department of Physical Therapy
University of Miami Miller School of Medicine
Coral Gables, Florida

Jackie H. Jones, EdD, MSN, RN
Assistant Professor of Nursing
Kennesaw State University
Kennesaw, Georgia

Lois S. Marshall, PhD, RN, CPN
Nurse Education Consultant, Independent
Nurse Researcher Scholar in Residence
Honor Society of Nursing, Sigma Theta Tau International
Indianapolis, Indiana

Tamika R. Sanchez-Jones, PhD, MBA, APRN, BC
John A. Hartford Foundation
Atlantic Philanthropies Claire M. Fagin Fellow
University of Iowa College of Nursing
Iowa City, Iowa

Ruth M. Tappen, EdD, RN, FAAN
Christine E. Lynn Eminent Scholar and Professor
Christine E. Lynn College of Nursing
Florida Atlantic University
Boca Raton, Florida

Theris A. Touhy, DNP, APRN, BC
Associate Professor
Christine E. Lynn College of Nursing
Florida Atlantic University
Boca Raton, Florida

Nancy E. Villanueva, PhD, ARNP, BC, CNRN
Nurse Practitioner—Neurosurgery
Jackson Memorial Hospital
Miami, Florida

Preface

The idea for this book was conceived in a discussion with Carol Davis, a colleague at the University of Miami. At the time, we were members of the Executive Committee of the Miami Area Geriatric Education Center (MAGEC) and had collaborated on many interdisciplinary projects. Carol is the author of *Patient Practitioner Interaction: An Experiential Manual for Developing the Art of Health Care, 4th ed.,* a wonderful book about communication for physical therapists and other health professionals. Carol encouraged me to write a book that would specifically address communication issues relevant to nurses. As a result of our collaboration, we were able to find common ground between her work on communication and my ideas about communication from a nursing perspective. I will always be grateful to her for her help and support in this project.

The response to the first edition of *Therapeutic Interaction in Nursing* was gratifying. Feedback from instructors and students described how helpful the content and the exercises have been in helping them to apply the principles to clinical situations. New chapters were written to address the needs identified by those in academic and clinical settings. Every chapter has been enhanced with current, evidence-based content, clinical examples, and exercises wherever relevant.

This book contains 14 chapters organized into three units. The first section, "Therapeutic Use of Self," contains two chapters. These introductory chapters give readers the opportunity to reflect on their life experiences and to relate them to the development of relationships with clients. Content on emotional and social intelligence is meant to help learners to recognize that their entire being is involved in relationships with clients.

This book can be used as a text by students taking a course in communication for nurses. It will be an excellent resource for students in an integrated curriculum or for nurses in a clinical setting. The first two sections ("Therapeutic Use of Self" and "Interacting with Others") will assist beginning students in preparing for the professional role and in focusing on the needs of clients rather than on their own anxiety or other needs.

The second section, "Interacting with Others," contains four chapters covering the helping interview and specific communication strategies. Cultural considerations that may affect communication are included. Readers identified a need for guidance on interaction with families. Because this content is relevant to most clinical situations, a chapter on interacting with families was added to this section.

The third section, "Communicating in Special Circumstances," has been enlarged and updated. The section includes chapters to correspond with special populations such as care of children, women in labor, older adults, clients with severe and persistent psychiatric illnesses, and individuals with cognitive impairment. Several chapters are new. Chapters on communication strategies to promote health literacy and communication with women in labor are generally not found in other books on communication.

The first two sections and the companion exercises will enhance learning for those who are beginning the clinical component of their nursing program, for individuals returning to nursing, or for people who are transitioning to a professional nursing program. Practicing nurses who are embarking on a career in psychiatric mental health nursing will find this content essential to their practice. Chapters in the third section can enhance student learning as they progress through the undergraduate curriculum. Specialty content will also be very relevant for nurses beginning careers or graduate programs with these populations. Specialty content and the companion exercises are excellent learning tools for those who are preparing for a certification examination.

Acknowledgments

I would like to acknowledge my former students and colleagues at the University of Miami School of Nursing and Health Studies for their support and suggestions during the process of revision. In particular, I would like to acknowledge Dr. Doris Ugarriza for her feedback on communication strategies for persons with psychiatric illnesses.

I am very grateful to my colleagues who wrote new chapters or updated existing chapters. Their efforts have increased the timeliness and relevance of this book.

I am especially grateful to Carol Davis who first suggested the idea to write this book. Her support has been very important to me, and her experience in writing about communication has been invaluable.

Many thanks to my students, patients, and research participants who have challenged me to communicate more effectively. I am also grateful to the members of the Miami Chapter of The Compassionate Friends, Inc., a support group for those who have experienced the death of a child, sibling, or grandchild. They have inspired me to communicate to the nursing community that we need to improve our skills when interacting with bereaved patients and families. A special thank you to Shelly Ellis who provided feedback on the chapter "Communicating at Times of Loss and Grief."

Finally, I am grateful to those who guide the next generation of nurses. The principles that are suggested in this book must be practiced. The learner's performance must be reviewed by supportive teachers, supervisors, and mentors.

Section 1
Therapeutic Use of Self

1

Understanding Ourselves and Our Relationships

Christine L. Williams, DNSc, APRN, BC and Carol M. Davis, DPT, EdD, MS, FAPTA

OBJECTIVES

1. To discuss the importance of self-awareness to effective helping

2. To analyze the interaction of the self and our relationships with others

3. To examine the development of a mature person as described by Erikson

4. To describe the role of childhood development in the formation of identity and self-esteem

It has been said that a nurse's most important tool is the therapeutic use of self. Our personalities and styles of relating have everything to do with how effectively we facilitate the healing process. If we were to ask nurses to assess their ability to relate effectively with people, few would admit to lapses in temper, irritability, or prejudice. Yet these and other negative behaviors can occur, especially when nurses lack self-awareness.

Although difficult to observe, behaviors such as lack of honesty and loyalty to one's colleagues and breaking confidences are common in health care. Often, nurses are unaware of their unprofessional behavior or the effect of their behavior on others. Clients challenge our sensitivity and maturity in unique ways. Clients react out of the stress of their illnesses or pain, but nurses must also work under stress. It requires great maturity and patience to respond in healing ways in less than ideal situations.

■ EMOTIONAL INTELLIGENCE

Because intelligence is multidimensional, cognitive or thinking intelligence is not enough to ensure that a nurse will be effective with patients. Another type of intelligence is necessary as well: emotional intelligence.[1] Emotional intelligence is the ability to notice, understand, and regulate one's emotions.[2] The nurse who can choose where, when, and how to express his or her emotions will avoid impulsive expression of potentially destructive emotions such as anger. Such self-awareness is essential to therapeutic interaction.

Emotional intelligence is important in another component of therapeutic interaction: the ability to understand emotions in others. Responding with compassion is possible when the nurse can see the hurt in an angry client's outburst or the fear in individuals who delay treatment until their condition becomes life threatening. Understanding the emotions that trigger behavior is fundamental to appreciating and caring for clients.[1]

Emotions cannot be separated from their neurobiological basis. LeDoux writes that there are two pathways from perceiving threat to action. One is a direct route through the emotional center of the brain, the amygdala. This kind of reaction is immediate and results in behavior on an emotional level without much thought. The other route is through the neocortex, the thinking part of the brain, where emotions are considered along with knowledge and experience. This slower, more thoughtful approach is likely to lead to rational behavior. When faced with a threat, the individual may react without thinking and come to regret those actions later. Therapeutic communication depends on the nurse's ability to react with thought as well as emotion to handle emotionally charged situations in a rational way.[3]

Emotional reactions have a powerful biological and psychological impact on other people. Our moods spread to others around us, especially those with whom we have close contact. Emotions of caring and compassion for our clients promote clients' trust and, in turn, facilitate our ability to promote client healing.

■ SOCIAL INTELLIGENCE

Noticing and regulating emotions in self and others is only a first step in becoming a competent helper. We need to use those abilities to develop effective relationships. Goleman[4] describes a person's interaction skill as his or her social intelligence. Nurses reveal their social intelligence in everyday clinical situations. Does the nurse treat the client respectfully, with dignity, and as an individual? A nurse's awareness of the client as a person is revealed at the most basic level with politeness and warmth in his or her interactions with the client. Social intelligence is conveyed by attentiveness to a client's needs. The client feels good when they are with you.

Examples of social intelligence at work include checking with the client to see if he or she needs pain medication, providing an explanation when a client is left waiting for an appointment, and providing comfort measures without being asked. Contrast this to nurses who perform tasks while barely noticing the person for whom the tasks are performed. For nurses, social intelligence goes beyond social skills. It includes treating the person as a person rather than an object.[4]

Our social aptitude will determine how effective we are in stressful situations. Imagine caring for a mother with a very sick child or a tearful adolescent in labor on a maternity unit. Are you confident that you can focus on the client's needs rather than your own discomfort? We provide compassionate care to clients who are suffering by knowing what they feel, understanding what they need, and wanting to help.[5] Self-awareness and life experience both play important roles in the process of coming to understand another person in need and interacting effectively to relieve their suffering.

In their review of research on suffering and caregiving,[5] Shulz and colleagues concluded that compassion had adverse effects on family caregivers' health. Nurses are also susceptible to the stresses of everyday exposure to clients who are suffering. The effect of helping on caregivers seems to be related to whether caregivers feel successful in reducing the care recipient's distress and whether they feel capable of meeting the caregiving challenge. Successful helping is very beneficial to mental and physical health. When caregivers are successful, they benefit from an increased sense of competence and self-esteem.[6]

■ INFLUENCE OF THE FAMILY ON SELF-ESTEEM

Each of us views the world from a unique perspective that we begin to develop as small children. Our worldview evolves out of what we hear and experience as children growing up in a unique family unit. Important adults, such as parents, close relatives, and teachers, influence us through their interactions.[7] Significant others guide children with tenderness when their behavior meets with their approval, or they redirect behaviors that fail to meet expectations. These learning experiences, combined with inborn characteristics, develop into a unique way of experiencing the world. Even twins growing up under the same circumstances will develop different views based upon which each chooses to notice.

Children are not little adults, as Piaget first clearly described.[8] Children have underdeveloped nervous systems and lack the capacity to move, think, and act in the same manner as adults. Children live in a land of make-believe, enjoy fantasy, and are egocentric. They are unable to handle abstract logic and are very present oriented and concrete. If you ask a child which of two parallel, identical pencils is longer, she or he will say, correctly, that both are the same length. But then if you slide one pencil so that it is ahead of the other, though still parallel, and then ask, "Which pencil is longer?" she or he will say the pencil that is ahead of the other is longer. In other words, children cannot conserve information. Likewise, children are unable to come outside of themselves and view themselves. Ask a child who has a brother if he has a brother and he'll say, "Yes." Ask him if his brother has a brother, he'll say, "No."[9]

Finally, children idolize their parents. They cope with feelings of helplessness and dependence by believing that their parents (or caregivers) are powerful and will protect them and care for them. Even when parents fail to protect them or meet their needs, most children continue to believe in them and will deny the negative experiences of the past.

Case example

Samuel experienced severe neglect from his mother, Claire, during his early years. When he was 10 years of age, they were separated for 6 months except for occasional supervised visits while Claire was treated for substance abuse in a long-term drug rehabilitation program. He was cared for by loving and attentive relatives. During the separation, he longed to be returned to his mother and looked forward to her visits with great excitement. He never referred to his suffering during those early years and seemed to remember only positive memories.

Erik Erikson[10] developed a useful description of the development of personality that centers on the successful resolution of tension in a series of steps encountered by the growing person from birth onward. A certain degree of accomplishment is required at each stage or the person will have to master those tasks later in life. Table 1-1 summarizes Erikson's theory of development. Case examples demonstrate how Erikson's stages can be applied to client situations.

Human beings are among few living creatures born without the capacity to obtain food independently. As infants, we must cry out to others around us to have our basic survival needs met. The fact that we are born totally dependent on others for our survival is a critical aspect of the development of our worldview. Who we are and our perceptions of the world depend on how others respond to us when we are helpless and what others say to us and about us. This is how our identity develops. It is obvious that the maturity of the parent and the extent to which the child is wanted and anticipated have a great deal to do with how the parent responds to the child and thus fosters or inhibits the development of a sense of self-identity and self-esteem.

Few of us grew up in ideal homes, but many of us have difficulty remembering the negative things about childhood. Remember that children idealize their parents. Adolescents give up those notions, but many replace them with strongly held traditions to honor and respect their parents. To idealize your parents is to idealize the way they raised you.[12] Part of maturation is to give up the idealized view of our parents and to replace it with a balanced awareness of their strengths and weaknesses. It is very important to look back at what was happening in

Table 1-1   Psychosocial Theory of Development: A Summary of Erikson's Stages of Development[10, 11]

Trust vs Mistrust (birth to 1 year)

Infants who receive consistent, tender care learn to trust. Because no caretaker is perfectly predictable and consistent, some mistrust does arise during infancy and continue throughout the life span. A person's ability to trust is related to the quality of care received during the first year of life. It is important to emerge from this stage with hope. Hope comes from more trust than mistrust. Predominance of mistrust will adversely affect relationships until positive life experiences help the person to develop more trust.

Case example

Sheryl, age 32, has been engaged to be married several times and has broken the engagements every time. Her relationships have been troubled since childhood and she has difficulty with trust. Sheryl's parents were drug addicts when she was an infant and she was raised by a variety of relatives. Life was usually unpredictable and she was never sure who to trust.

Autonomy vs Shame and Doubt (2 to 4 years)

Toddlers begin to experiment with autonomy or independence. They discover that they can hold on to people and things or they can let go or push them away. They can say "No!" and they often do! Their growing biological independence promotes feelings of autonomy. Shame comes from the realization that they can make mistakes and be judged. Doubt arises when the child

Case example

Throughout his early years, Jack, age 46, was rarely rewarded for independent action. His parents were controlling and perfectionists. They criticized him constantly. Now he finds it difficult to take risks at work. He sees others being promoted and earning higher salaries, yet his fear of making mistakes and his severe reactions to criticism keep him from being more successful.

Table 1-1   Psychosocial Theory of Development (continued)

realizes that he or she is not completely independent. To emerge from this stage with a sense of will, the child must experience more autonomy than shame and doubt. For autonomy and will to prevail, children need experiences with sensitive adults who encourage their growing independence and redirect their problematic behavior without harsh criticism.

Initiative vs Guilt (4 to 5 years)

At this stage children become aware of sexuality and sex roles. They become interested in competing with one parent for the love of the other parent. Have you ever noticed a young child trying to squeeze between their parents on the couch? Healthy parents communicate their love for their child while demonstrating that the child cannot really come between them. As children learn to restrict their competitive behaviors to more socially acceptable outlets, they develop self-control and the capacity for guilt. Children at this age are ready to channel their ambitions by playing, learning, communicating, and competing with peers. Adults react to the child's initiatives with approval or disapproval. As adults encourage children to engage in socially acceptable pursuits and approve of their imaginative play, they foster a sense of purpose and minimize guilt and inhibition.

> **Case example**
>
> Stacey, age 24, grew up with parents who took an active interest in her developing imagination. Her mother posted her artistic creations around the house and praised her for cooperative play with peers. When her curiosity and exuberance led her to infringe on the rights of others, her parents gently redirected her to other pursuits. Stacey has a clear sense of purpose in her life and confidence in her ability to succeed.

Industry vs Inferiority (6 to 11 years)

The school age years bring children into contact with other adults such as teachers, coaches, and other adults in the community. Their contacts with peers increase through school and other activities. These experiences provide the opportunity to develop cognitive and social skills. They also learn skills that will help them to be successful at work such as showing up on time, organization, attention to detail, and perseverance. If they find that their efforts are rewarded with approval, they develop a sense of industry and competence. If they receive disapproval regardless of effort, they develop feelings of inferiority instead. Children can be rejected for factors outside their control (e.g., race, religion, poverty), and these experiences can result in feelings of inferiority.

> **Case example**
>
> Tom grew up in an urban neighborhood plagued by poverty and crime. His mother worked long hours and had little time to encourage him to do well at school. Most of the families in the neighborhood expected little from their children. When he went to school, Tom felt inferior to his peers who had money for designer clothes and social activities. A teacher took an interest in his artistic talents and helped him to develop a sense of competence at school.

Identity vs Role Confusion (12 to 18 years)

Sexual and aggressive drives become active during adolescence. These strong feelings propel children toward seeking relationships with others. They worry about how they appear to others. Will they be accepted? What

Table 1-1   Psychosocial Theory of Development (continued)

groups do they want to find acceptance from? All this questioning leads to the ultimate questions: Who am I? What am I good at? The adolescent tries out different identities. As part of the pursuit of uniqueness and independence, adolescents often choose identities that bring negative reactions from parents. These actions are generally temporary if they are not reinforced. Being part of a group of peers is very important to the development of an identity. Finding an identity enables one to practice fidelity or commitment to a way of life.

Intimacy vs Isolation (19 to 34)

With a firm sense of who they are, young adults are freer from self-absorption and ready to find intimacy. They are now able to focus more on what a partner wants and needs than on how they appear to the potential partner. The challenge for young adults is to learn to be emotionally intimate with a partner without giving up one's separate identity. Sexual intimacy is not enough to accomplish this task. A firm sense of identity is necessary to make emotional intimacy possible. Without identity the young adult may find the task of emotional intimacy too frightening. Failure to achieve this task results in loneliness and isolation.

Generativity vs Stagnation (35 to 60)

When adults are comfortable in their ability to develop and sustain intimacy with a partner, they can focus on caring for others and helping the next generation. Adults achieve generativity in many ways. The obvious way is to have children and to "give back" by helping them to grow and develop. Adults can also "give" to the next generation by mentoring others at work, teaching, or becoming involved in causes that improve the environment or the wider world. Stagnation occurs when the adult remains self-absorbed. This can occur whether or not one is a parent.

Integrity vs Despair (60 to death)

In late life, adults struggle with accepting themselves and question the meaning of their lives. Was my life meaningful? Am I at peace with my decisions? Am I satisfied with my relationships, what I achieved or failed to achieve? If they are satisfied with the answers to these self-examinations, they can face death with integrity. If not, they experience bitterness, depression, and despair.

Case example

Marcia, a college student, was close to failing in school. She changed her major three times and was afraid that she wouldn't be able to decide on a career choice. She shocked her parents when she dropped out of school to travel and to "find herself." During her year of travel and odd jobs, she was able to come to a decision and commit to a career. She returned to school with a better sense of her identity and was successful in her course work.

Case example

Ingrid and Alberto, ages 22 and 23, are young adults in love. They frequently argue and defend their separate identities and their "rights" in the relationship. Gradually they become more comfortable with taking risks to share their vulnerabilities without fear of rejection or of being overwhelmed by the other. They begin to make plans for a committed relationship.

Case example

Mitch, age 50, has been addicted to cocaine throughout adulthood and exemplifies stagnation. His relationship with his ex-wife and children is strained, and he rarely sees them. He has had a troubled employment history and spends much of his time in crisis.

Case example

Samuel Chase is 90 years old and hospitalized for pneumonia. Despite his nurse's attempts to make him comfortable, he complains constantly. He is irritable and verbally abusive. He doesn't have visitors, which is no surprise to the staff. They find it difficult to respond to him with empathy. He exemplifies despair.

Source: Adapted from Ramsden, E. (1986). Affective dimensions in client care. In O. Payton (Ed.), *Psychosocial aspects of clinical practice.* New York: Churchill Livingstone.

your family when you were growing up as one way to increase your awareness of your self and your worldview.

Each child is born into a complex family situation and encounters various challenges, as described by Erikson, as he or she develops day-by-day. If a child is born to parents who experience physical comfort, emotional calm, and joy in his or her presence, the child will develop a sense of trust and a view that the world is a warm and loving place. If, however, the child is a burden to the parents, he or she will come to believe that the world is uncertain. A child born to a family with violent parents will experience the world as a hostile place and will learn to mistrust others. In fact, painful childhood memories are stored in the brain even when we have limited ability to describe them in words. These memories continue to affect our behavior as adults until we become more aware of them and replace them with positive experiences.[1]

It is unrealistic to expect a person to complete each stage of development on schedule without any difficulties. Individuals may have partial resolution of a developmental task at times or may be unsuccessful at other times. The degree of success with a stage of development will influence the person's ability to successfully complete the next stage. Adults may still be working on developmental tasks from childhood because they were unable to complete them successfully at the time. Parents use their own experience to guide their children through these tasks. If their own experiences were less than successful, their ability to parent will be similarly affected. Generally, adults who do not parent well were, themselves, not parented well. Dysfunctional parents learn to be dysfunctional from the families in which they grew up.

How we respond to the world today is influenced by our biological attributes, past experiences, sense of ourselves, and the adequacy of our self-esteem. The development of healthy self-esteem requires more successful than unsuccessful resolution of the tensions described by Erikson either as we mature or later. As adults, we can examine our growing up experiences, gain insight into our dysfunctional views, and consciously change our distorted worldview to give us a more accurate focus of the world and of ourselves.

■ HEALTHY OR OPEN FAMILIES

Healthy families interact in ways that have been described as "open" in contrast to the "closed" functioning

---

Case example

Sara is the 22-year-old mother of 18-month-old Cami. Cami is a healthy, active toddler who loves to run and is unaware of dangerous situations in the environment. Sara enjoys taking Cami to the park where she meets other young mothers with their children. Sara's ideas about parenting are based on the way she was parented. She expects Cami to obey her when she commands her to "Stop running!" or to come to her when she calls her name. When Cami looks back at her mother, laughs, and keeps running, Sara is enraged and slaps her to communicate her disapproval. Sara cannot understand why her daughter continues to "disobey," and Cami cannot understand why her mother withdraws her approval. Cami is learning to be distrustful and doubtful about her growing independence.

---

of troubled or dysfunctional families (Table 1-2). A family functions to provide a safe and supportive environment for all of its members to learn basic values, grow, and become more fully human. In healthy families, members feel empowered to adapt to change and supported in coping with the stresses of the world both outside the home and within. The stress inside the home is usually perceived to be less than the stress faced outside in the world except in transient phases of family crisis.

In healthy families, individuals are recognized as being unique and having worth. There is open communication in which members feel free to speak their opinion but do so with concern and caring for others. In sum, family members feel safe, supported, encouraged, and appreciated. Roles and responsibilities of family members are flexible but clear. People function well day-to-day and in crisis. Finally, quality time is shared by parents and children and is enjoyed.[13]

■ DYSFUNCTIONAL OR CLOSED FAMILIES

Charles Whitfield believes that many people grow up in families that stifle the development of the true self and instead cultivate in the child a false or "codependent" self.[14] Children need to feel as if they are safe and protected at all times. They need to feel free to ask questions, run and play, and know the boundaries that parents set for them are fair and consistent. Children need to feel as if they can be children, learning and growing without fear of being ridiculed or punished cruelly for making

Table 1-2 Characteristics of Families

Open/Healthy	Troubled	Closed/Unhealthy
Open to change Flexible responses to each situation	Nothing can be done What's the use?	Rigid, fixed, harsh rules Right vs wrong, no exceptions
High self-worth People are valued as individuals	Shaky self-worth Cover feelings of low self-control	Evasive responses Low self-worth, shaming behavior Low ownership—blaming
Functional defenses Use defenses as a coping skill with insight	Use defenses to hide pain Defenses more often deny real feelings *Choice is lost* Always smile, cry, complain, etc.	No choice—react compulsively and rigidly out of fear Short fuses Avoidance or rage
Clear rules discussed: hours, respect for property, telephone use, chores, etc. Rules are regularly negotiated	Unclear—rules are inconsistent Depends on who is asked what day, which child, etc.	Edicts or no rules at all Chaos—rules cannot be followed
People take risks to express feelings, ideas, beliefs	Not safe to express feelings or give opinions: "Don't rock the boat" Can't disagree	Denial of problems Ignore bizarre behaviors No talk rule—even about serious problems, especially drinking, drugs
Can deal with stress, pick up on others' pain Nurturing and caring for each other Seek out those in pain to support, encourage	Avoid pain Do not see it in others Sweep problems under the rug Pretend all is okay	Denial of stress Can't cope with any more—glazed eyes don't see pain Ignore basic need to be seen, acknowledged Children become early helpers
Accepts life stages, welcomes them Celebrate growth—sexuality, new friends, accomplishments	Parents may compete with children—growth is accepted painfully—don't talk about sex Try to keep children dependent	Passage of time is ignored Change is feared—adults are treated as children, children may try to act like adults Children are ridiculed, teased but try to become helpful
Either clear hierarchy or egalitarian—strong parental coalition Less need to control Can negotiate	Hidden coalitions across generations Parental coalition is weak—rigid or shifting pattern of domination	Either upside down family—children may run it—or chaotic No giving out of rules, or one parent is in charge of all and can't cope
Affect is open Direct expression of feelings—all feelings are okay Anger is in context of awareness of other person Considerate of others	Negativism, low feeling, bickering, argumentative, controlled mood, some feelings are okay, some not Inconsistent acceptance of feelings	Cynicism, open hostility, violence, sadism—actually try to manipulate and hurt each other Only happiness is allowed

Source: Reprinted with permission from SLACK Incorporated: Davis, C.M. (2006). *Patient Practitioner Interaction: An Experimental Manual for Developing the Art of Health Care* (4th ed.). Thorofare, NJ: SLACK Incorporated.

mistakes. Children need to be invited to feel their feelings and put them into words so they can learn how not to be impulsive or controlled by their feelings.

Dysfunctional families, however, respond to the dependence of a child in ways that interfere with their development. In the dysfunctional family, children do not feel free to make mistakes, but they feel that if they are not "right" they will be harshly criticized. In such a family, children receive approval when they are compliant, considerate, and unselfish.[14] Adults may be too authoritarian, determined to break the child's will at any cost, or they may be unavailable due to extreme circumstances such as war, poor health of the parent, or escape behavior such as alcoholism and other addictions, work, mental illness, or travel. Children, who think of their parents as perfect, soon begin realizing that they are not free to be a child. They may adopt another way of being, usually that of parenting the parent and/or raising younger siblings. As a result, a false self emerges in the child. According to psychologist Alice Miller,[15] the persistent denial of the true self and true feelings takes its toll in the development of coping mechanisms and a realistic view of the world.

■ HEALTH PROFESSIONAL'S SELF-ESTEEM

It has been said that many people enter the health professions for a variety of reasons. We seek opportunities for generativity, to feel important and respected, or to be needed. Some of the less flattering reasons include a need to be depended upon, a need to control people, and a need to get one's natural attention and affection needs met. Some may be looking for emotional healing themselves by making life easier for others. Few people are conscious of these motives, however. Nonetheless, some health professionals act in ways that are responsive to their emotions and do things that are, in the long run, harmful to clients and contrary to the healing process. These are the characteristics of *early helpers.*

Dysfunctional families often create children who can be described as early helpers. One example of a dysfunctional family is that in which one or both parents are addicted to alcohol. Millions of Americans grew up or are presently living in families affected by addiction.[16] The literature that has developed from the Adult Children of Alcoholics (ACOA) movement in the United States has shed needed light on the distorted worldview of the adult who grew up in a home in which one or more parents were unable or unwilling

to parent. This circumstance encourages the development of the "false self," stifles the successful resolution of the tensions described by Erikson, and contributes to chronic low self-esteem and feelings of not being "good enough."[13] All children experience shame, but children in dysfunctional families take on shame as part of their identity. Children in dysfunctional families are never free to be children; they have to be grown-up and helpful. Because this is indeed a difficult task, they feel that they are always doing something wrong. Shame is different from guilt. Whitfield[14] describes shame as "the uncomfortable or painful feeling that we experience when we realize that part of us is defective, bad, incomplete, rotten, phony, inadequate, or a failure." Thus, guilt says, "I made a mistake"; shame says, "I am a mistake."

Self-esteem can be viewed as the extent to which we are able and willing to believe in our essential goodness in the face of our own lack of perfection. More than simply self-acceptance, self-esteem includes pride in the promise of ongoing growth and change with maturity, the hope of a richer, more peaceful and congruent life as a result of honest, day-to-day struggle. Children reared in dysfunctional families feel the shame of never being quite good enough rather than confidence and pride in doing the best they can. When feelings of shame are identified and replaced with a more realistic view of our imperfections and essential goodness, self-acceptance becomes possible.

Parental dysfunction may result from many causes. The critical factor seems to be how well the parent was present for the growing child in such a way as to encourage the natural curiosity of the child, the natural desire to learn, grow, and explore the world, how well the parent nurtured and protected the child, and how safe and free from potential harm the child felt.[14] When the parent is unable to assume those responsibilities, for whatever reason, the child starts parenting the parent, and an early helper emerges. A common description given by children from dysfunctional families is that they feel that they were a burden; they feel that they were being bad when they simply showed natural curiosity or asked questions. In fact, it was their very existence that seemed to bring discomfort to their family.

Children are not meant to be parents. When they take on this role, they take on a false self, and authentic feelings of curiosity, fear, and need become repressed, covered by feigned feelings of bravery and affection in an attempt to please the parent. Common characteristics that materialize from the distorted worldview and false view of the self include:

- Fear of losing control

- Fear of feelings that seem overwhelming

- Fear of conflict

- Fear of abandonment

- Fear of becoming alcoholic or drug dependent

- Fear of becoming dependent on another person for survival

- Overdeveloped sense of responsibility

- Feelings of guilt and grief

- Inability to relax and have fun spontaneously

- Harsh self-criticism

- A tendency to lie, even when it is not "necessary"

- A tendency to let one's mind wander, to lose track of a conversation, to figuratively "leave the room"

- Denial and/or the tendency to create reality the way you want it to be rather than the way it is

- Difficulties getting close to people, difficulties with intimacy

- Feelings of vulnerability, of being a victim in a harsh world

- Compulsive behavior, tendency to become addicted to things that alter mood

- Comfort with taking charge in a crisis; panic if you cannot "do" something in a crisis

- Confusion between love and pity

- Black and white perspective—all good or all bad

- Internalizing—taking responsibility for others' problems

- Tendency to react rather than act

- Experiencing stress-related illnesses

- Overachievement

Children from dysfunctional families are sometimes the "heroes" in health care, the ones who, at great personal sacrifice, go above and beyond the call to fix things for everyone else and are praised and admired for it. They thrive on rescuing others and on creating order out of chaos.

■ THE NEED TO KNOW OURSELVES

The nurse must know him- or herself well; he or she must be aware of behaviors that will result in harmful dependence on clients for meeting personal needs for intimacy. The end goal of all healing is the restoration of independent function for the highest and deepest quality of life possible for the client. We encourage clients to make it on their own. Nurses must be vigilant to avoid depending on our clients to meet our needs for attention, affection, and/or power and authority.

Self-awareness helps us to identify our emotions and to monitor our own behavior. It is very difficult to help others if we need help ourselves. Help is widely available through counseling, participation in support groups and psychotherapy groups, and in 12-step programs such as Al Anon, Overeaters Anonymous, Alcoholics Anonymous, Gamblers Anonymous, and Adult Children of Alcoholics (ACOA), all of which can be found throughout the United States and in other countries. The goal of seeking help is always to become acquainted with the true self and to gain self-acceptance.

■ CONCLUSION

A lack of self-understanding can interfere with helping others, therefore, taking the time to reflect on your past as well as your present life is a crucial part of a career in nursing. Becoming familiar with your strengths and vulnerabilities will help you to minimize inappropriate emotional reactions and maximize thoughtful, compassionate responses to the needs of clients. Developing self-understanding and learning to use your emotions to enhance relationships will be a lifelong process. Caring for people of different backgrounds and in a variety of life experiences will forever challenge you to grow personally.

REFERENCES

1. Goleman, D. (1995). *Emotional intelligence.* New York: Bantam Books.

2. Schutte, N.S., Malouff, J.M., Bobik, C., Coston, T.D., Geeson, C., Rhodes, E., et al. (2001). Emotional intelligence and interpersonal relations. *The Journal of Social Psychology, 141*(4), 523–536.

3. LeDoux, J. (1996). *The emotional brain.* New York: Touchstone.

4. Goleman, D. (2006). *Social intelligence.* New York: Bantam Books.

5. Shulz, R., Hebert, R.S., Dew, M.A., Brown, S.L., Scheier, M.F., Beach, S.R., et al. (2007). Patient suffering and caregiver compassion: New opportunities for research, practice, and policy. *The Gerontologist, 47*, 1, 4–13.

6. Post, S.G. (2005). Altruism, happiness and health: It's good to be good. *International Journal of Behavioral Medicine, 12*(2), 66–77.

7. Sullivan, H.S. (1954). *The interpersonal theory of psychiatry.* New York: WW Norton & Company.

8. Piaget, J. (1954). *The construction of reality in the child.* New York: Basic Books.

9. Bradshaw, J. (1988). *Bradshaw on: The family.* Deerfield Beach, FL: Health Communications, Inc.

10. Erikson, E.H. (1968). *Identity, youth and crisis.* New York: WW Norton.

11. Crain, W. (1980). Chapter 12. Erikson and the eight stages of life. *Theories of development: Concepts and applications.* Englewood Cliffs, NJ: Prentice Hall.

12. Rogers, C.R. (1961). *On becoming a person.* Boston: Houghton Mifflin Company.

13. Department of Health and Human Services. (1990). *Identifying successful families: An overview of constructs and selected resources.* Washington, DC.

14. Whitfield, C.L. (1986). *Healing the child within.* Baltimore: The Resource Group.

15. Miller, A. (1981). *The drama of the gifted child.* New York: Basic Books.

16. Grant, B.F., Dawson, D.A., Stinson, F.S., Chou, S.P., Dufour, M.C., Pickering, R.P. (2004). The 12-month prevalence and trends in DSM-IV alcohol abuse and dependence: United States, 1991–1992, and 2001–2002. *Drug and Alcohol Dependence, 74*, 223–234.

EXERCISES

1. Self-Assessment

In a spiral notebook that you can keep confidential, answer each of the following questions as honestly as you can for this moment. It is suggested that you use a notebook so that you can save these reflections and refer back to them later. Allow at least half a page for each question. Jot down the first thing that comes to mind for each question, then take additional time to express your thoughts clearly. You may wish to complete the entire set over a period of a week or so, taking one or two questions at a time. When you have completed these exercises, share your conclusions with a trusted friend or confidant.

A. Who am I?
   Date:

   1. I would describe myself physically as . . .

   2. I would describe my personality as . . .

   3. Others would describe me as . . .

   4. When I think about who I am, I am most proud of . . .

   5. I was most ashamed of . . .

   6. I get angriest when . . .

   7. I'm most anxious that . . .

   8. When I am nervous I usually . . .

   9. People are essentially (good, bad, neutral) . . .

  10. Characteristics of other people that impress me most include . . .

  11. Goals I want to achieve:

     a. With this course . . .

     b. In my lifetime . . .

Discussion

When you have answered these questions, write a description about yourself from what you have discovered. Are you totally happy with yourself at this point? What would you change? What did you learn about yourself that will assist you in being a health professional? What may detract from your effectiveness?

B.   What about my family of origin (those who raised me)?

    1. If I were to use one word to describe my family (as a whole) it would be . . .

    2. The best thing about growing up in my family was . . .

    3. The most challenging part of growing up in my family was . . .

    4. In my family, disagreements were . . .

    5. In my family, talking about a problem was . . .

Discussion

When you have answered these questions, summarize what you have learned about your family of origin. How have you learned to relate to others? In what ways will your experiences affect how you relate with clients?

2. Journal

In your self-assessment notebook, begin a journal about yourself. Most of us confuse the concept of a journal with a diary. A diary is designed to record significant events in one's life. A journal is a letter to yourself designed to stimulate reflection about an experience rather than just recording the experience. One way to keep from simply recording the event is to begin each entry with the following phrases:

    What I felt during the exercise.

    What I learned about myself.

    So what? Significance or meanings of my learning.

    Your journal should be kept in a book with a cover on pages that do not easily become dislodged. Entries are to be written following each chapter. Many find it useful to journal as a way of privately discussing the chapter and its personal significance. Your journal is what you make it. Most people are unaccustomed to this sort of activity, however, and some dislike writing. For a short time, make a commitment to this activity. Remember, this journal is by you, for your personal use. Set aside the time on your calendar, and when you get into the routine of it, it will become rewarding.

3. Family Genogram

A genogram is a map of a family for several generations. It is a very useful picture that reveals patterns. An example of a genogram is shown below. Different symbols are used to represent male and female members of the family as well as type and quality of the relationships.

    Draw a diagram of your family (your family genogram) for at least three generations. Label anything that seems important to you. A genogram is a way to display relationships within a family across generations.

What patterns emerge? What do you now know about yourself that you failed to see before? What stories are important enough to be handed down? Who or what is the family proud of? What secrets does the family hide from others?

Perhaps questions came up for you about various family members' lives and habits. Write to relatives asking them to fill in the missing pieces to help you better understand your heritage. Try to locate pictures from long ago of yourself with other family members.

Journal about your feelings and awareness from this exercise. Can you identify behaviors that you have developed from your family that may interfere with helping others? Comment on any and problem solve ways in which you might be able to work through those behaviors.

Figure 1-1 Family Genogram

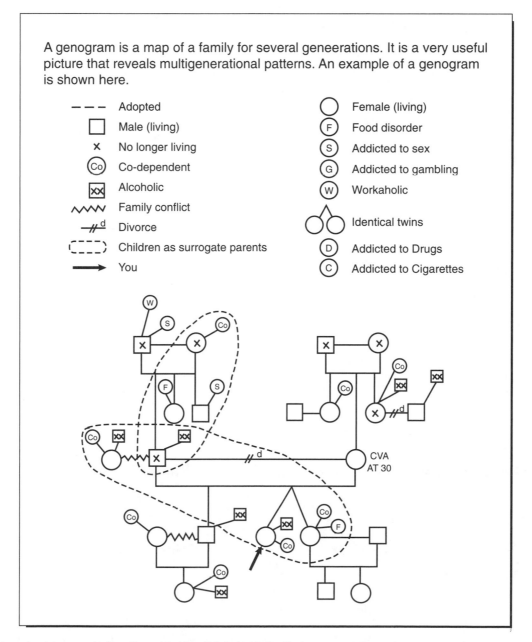

Source: Reprinted with permission from Davis, C.M. (2006). *Patient practitioner interaction: An experiential manual for developing the art of health care* (4th Ed.). Thorofare, NJ: SLACK Incorporated.

2

Using the Self to Promote Health

Christine L. Williams, DNSc, APRN, BC and Carol M. Davis, DPT, EdD, MS, FAPTA

OBJECTIVES

1. To consider the purpose of helping

2. To explore the behaviors that promote or interfere with effective helping

3. To describe some of the characteristics of therapeutic communication

4. To distinguish empathy from related interpersonal interactions

5. To reveal the characteristics of effective helpers

Nurses assist clients to achieve their health-related goals including improving their relationships with others. Using intentionality, nurses work with clients to promote health when possible or, at the end of life, to promote a peaceful death. Each encounter with a client, regardless of how brief, is an important opportunity to develop a healing relationship. (*Intentionality* is defined as focused awareness accessing universal life energy in the present moment to promote client well-being and healing.)[1] Therapeutic communication is an integral part of the nurse–patient relationship. It involves commitment and caring.[2] It helps us to transcend the "doing" that is characteristic of task-focused nursing and to participate in the important tasks of "being" including finding meaning in our relationships with clients.[1] The help that nurses offer to their clients is much more than technical expertise. The relationship between nurse and client is a powerful healing force by itself. This chapter focuses on the general nature of effective communication in the helping process.

Hildegard Peplau,[3] the "mother of psychiatric nursing" wrote that "nursing is a human relationship between an individual who is sick or in need of health services and a nurse especially educated to recognize and to respond to the need for help." Peplau also wrote that nursing is both educative and therapeutic. Every interaction between a nurse and a client includes a learning experience for the client about relationships—helping relationships in particular. If the client experiences a collaborative relationship with the nurse in which he or she is accepted and valued, the result will be personal growth and development. The client will be strengthened and better able to meet similar crises in the future.

Effective helping involves identifying opportunities for growth as well as problems. As nurses, we bring important knowledge and skills and offer them to clients who need help to understand their health and to act in ways that promote health. We provide the conditions for our clients to identify their goals and then help them to meet those goals.

Therapeutic communication, or the use of verbal and nonverbal messages to establish a therapeutic relationship, is also essential to the use of the self as an instrument of healing. Therapeutic communication will be explained in greater detail in this chapter and throughout this book.

How you view yourself will markedly affect your communication with clients. Remember that your self-concept affects the way you view the world and the way you communicate. Most of us have felt the discomfort of interacting with a person who continually apologizes for him- or herself, who distorts what we say, or who responds

17

with negativity and self-contempt. Each of us holds opinions and ideas about ourselves, but our essential self-worth forms the core around which those ideas merge. Negative self-worth is the most important factor that nurses must change in themselves to communicate from a healing perspective.

To develop your role as an effective, compassionate communicator, observe people around you. Are there nurses who you think of as role models? Observe their communication styles and the reactions they receive from their clients. How would you characterize their interactions? How do they balance the demands of nursing tasks with presence and communication with clients? Are they satisfied with their role as nurses? Positive role models can challenge each of us to continue to develop our skills in relating to clients.

Nurse–patient relationships have been described over and over in the nursing literature.[4] Assumptions underlying effective helping relationships in nursing include that the relationship must be

- linear—allowing for progression through orientation, working, and termination phases;

- based on client trust;

- enduring in time;

- cooperative (welcomed by clients who are willing to collaborate with nurses).[4]

Although these characteristics may be an ideal that nurses have come to expect, we will not always meet these expectations. In reality, nurses help clients even when the nurse–patient relationship is brief. It may involve one encounter that may last only minutes. Some nurse–patient relationships do not involve trust. Clients are sometimes uncooperative or even rejecting. Psychiatric nurses often encounter these conditions in their work with psychotic patients. In even the most challenging relationships, nurses can assist clients toward meeting their health-related goals. We can make the most of each interaction to provide care, healing, and comfort.

When the client's and nurse's expectations about the relationship differ, there is decreased client and nurse satisfaction. One example is the nurse who expects to be in control and the client who expects to be self-reliant. Nurses who are accustomed to a position of authority may insist on relating as an authority figure and rely on giving advice as a strategy for helping. Clients who are placed in a relatively powerless position will feel dependent and helpless. Many adults will feel resentful rather than grateful. Such interactions are troubling for both the client and the nurse. No person can take responsibility for another person. We can only take responsibility for ourselves. Sometimes clients do not have the ability to be in charge of their own lives—small children or adults who are unconscious, for example. Even then, we consider the perspective of the family.

Another example of a troubled interaction is the nurse who has a need to be told how helpful or even how irreplaceable he or she is to the client. In this case, the client's needs become secondary and the nurse loses effectiveness. We cannot expect clients to meet our needs for approval and belonging.

Clients may come to us for many reasons, but the key questions remain: What are the health issues from the client's perspective? And what are the client's goals in the healing process? How can we partner with the client/family to resolve their health issues? Therapeutic communication is a strategy that supports the development of effective partnerships.

■ THERAPEUTIC COMMUNICATION

Certain identifiable elements characterize therapeutic or healing communication. In the nurse–client interaction, the nurse:

- Is fully present—Is totally focused on the client and his or her ideas about the situation. Does not get preoccupied with the client's past or future or in the nurse's own problems. Allows interaction with the client to command the nurse's full attention.

- Listens—Listens with the whole self to ascertain the client's meanings and goals. Clarifies interpretations of what is heard. Resists categorizing or projecting personal beliefs and values. Resists giving quick advice or telling the client what to do.

- Speaks—Communicates hope not just with an expression of ideas but with the ability to express those ideas from inner conviction to outer clarity. Self-awareness enables the nurse to articulate well thought-out ideas regarding the role of the client in the healing process.

- Honors the client's autonomy—Asks questions to ascertain the truth about the situation as the client perceives it. Communicates that the client is worth listening to, that he or she has important information to add to this process. Conveys expertise, maintains confidentiality and informed consent.[1,5,7]

Thus, the therapeutic use of oneself includes communication that places the client in a position of informed equal, inevitably responsible for any positive outcomes in the helping process.

■ A Closer Look at Interpersonal Interaction

A key element of therapeutic communication is having an *attitude of respect* for the client. Respect includes a nonjudgmental approach and a belief that the client is capable of learning and growing. Ultimately, clients are entitled to manage their own lives in a way that is best for them. As obvious as this may seem, it is not always easy to have a nonjudgmental attitude. This attitude of acceptance can be quite challenging when one disapproves of the client's behavior. Approving of the client's behavior is not the same as acceptance. It is not necessary to approve. It is possible to understand why the client has made certain life choices. For example, a client may be involved in an illegal activity and was raised in an environment where this activity was commonplace. It is still possible to respect the dignity and worth of this client as a person despite disagreeing with his or her lifestyle choices or behaviors. The nurse can practice being nonjudgmental by giving undivided attention when listening and by refraining from offering advice. Suspending judgment is facilitated by purposefully viewing the situation from the client's point of view.

There are several possible interpersonal processes within the nurse–client relationship that must be understood.

Sympathy involves having similar feelings about something. If the nurse is in agreement with the client's feelings, the nurse experiences sympathy. The nurse can feel joyful about the client's success or feel sadness about the client's bad news. This is sympathy, or "fellow feeling." It is very commonly felt in health care and it is appropriate in the healing relationship with clients.[5,6]

Pity, on the other hand, rarely, if ever, is appropriate. When a nurse pities a client, he or she feels sympathy with condescension. "You poor thing," conveys an inappropriate inequality between the nurse and the client. It demeans the personhood of the client. Pity may draw us to help others, but to help with condescension gives the message to the client that the nurse is judging him or her to be "pitiful."[5,6]

Identification can interfere with healing communication as well. When the nurse identifies with the client, he or she begins to feel at one with the client. In that process, he or she may lose sight of their differences. For example, just because the nurse and client both have the same last name or both come from similar backgrounds does not mean that they do not have different values about health care. The nurse may assume that the client wants to know everything there is to know about a disease or disorder because that is what the nurse would want. The nurse may project his or her values onto the client and act in ways that make the client less important or less relevant to the healing process.[5,6]

Empathy is always helpful in a therapeutic relationship. Empathy involves thinking about or perceiving a situation from the client's perspective as well as sensing the client's feelings in that situation.[5] To experience empathy, the nurse creates a healing presence. The stresses of the day are put aside and all of the nurse's enthusiasm, energy, and attentiveness are directed toward the client's inner experience. At the same time, the nurse maintains objectivity and enlists his or her experience, knowledge, and skills to respond in a caring, hopeful manner. When the nurse feels empathy, the client feels understood.[5,6]

Empathy takes place in three overlapping stages (Figure 2-1). The first stage is the cognitive stage of focusing on the other. We listen carefully in an attempt to put ourselves in the place of the other. The second stage, following just a millisecond after, is, by far, the most significant. This is the "crossing over" stage wherein we feel ourselves crossing over for a moment into the frame of reference or the lived world of the other person. We feel so at one with the other that we forget momentarily that we are two separate beings. This is the identification stage of empathy.[5,6] The third stage resolves the temporary confusion as we come back into our "own skin" and feel a special alignment with the other after having experienced the crossing over.[7] This third stage resembles sympathy or "fellow feeling." Thus, empathy can be described as a momentary merging with another person in a unique moment of shared meaning.[5,6]

When empathy occurs, nurses need not lose their therapeutic objectivity by getting too close to their clients. Instead, what is experienced is a healing presence that allows the client and nurse to remain fully separate in the healing process. It is when the process stops at identification that we lose our objectivity and our effectiveness. Thus, empathy is

Figure 2-1   Three Stages of Empathy

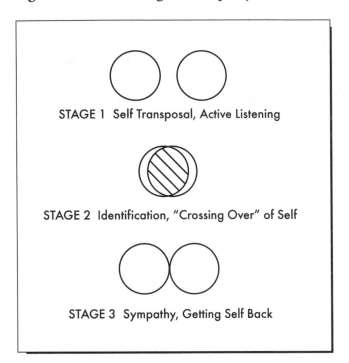

STAGE 1 Self Transposal, Active Listening

STAGE 2 Identification, "Crossing Over" of Self

STAGE 3 Sympathy, Getting Self Back

an interpersonal process that, among other things, empowers us to communicate therapeutically with clients, thus contributing to the therapeutic relationship.

To experience empathy, it is important that the nurse feels secure and peaceful. If the nurse feels threatened, empathy will be less likely to occur. During a threat, there are neurochemical changes in the brain that actually interfere with the experience of empathy. When the brain prepares for fight or flight, opioids or powerful pain relieving neurochemicals are released. These neurochemicals have a numbing effect on pain (and emotions), which is very helpful in situations involving physical danger. In situations involving emotional threat, this numbing may block the nurse's ability to empathize.[8] This helps explain why nurses who are stressed or experiencing "burn out" seem to feel so little compassion or caring for clients. When this happens, the solution is to reduce the nurse's sense of threat so that he or she is able to feel again.

■ LEVELS OF INTIMACY IN PROFESSIONAL INTERACTION

The challenge, then, is for the nurse to develop and maintain a therapeutic relationship with the client for the purpose of promoting health. Nurses may be drawn to clients who are easy to talk to and who meet the nurse's need for

appreciation and gratitude. If a relationship is to be therapeutic, it is imperative that this relationship remain focused on the goal of promoting client health and healing. How does the nurse foster trust and reveal humanness without allowing the relationship to change into a more involved friendship or social relationship? Revealing too many details about oneself might confuse the client by seeming to convey that the nurse is willing to give more than is appropriate for the helping process or that the nurse wants help solving his or her own problems. Powell[9] describes five different levels of communication that one can use as guidelines for communicating effectively without revealing too much. These levels lie on a continuum from near indifference to extreme intimacy:

- Level five: Cliché conversation—No genuine human sharing takes place. "How are you?" "It's nice to see you." Cliché conversation protects people from each other and prevents the likelihood of meaningful communication.

- Level four: Reporting facts—Almost nothing personal is revealed. Some sharing takes place about information such as diagnostic data or the weather.

- Level three: Personal ideas and judgments—Some information about oneself is shared, often in response to the client's conversation. Topics talked about often relate to the client's illness or the process the client is going through.

- Level two: Feelings and emotions—A deep trust is required to share this level, and if a person fears judgment, it will be impossible to relate at this level. Caring requires this level of communication. Each person wants to be deeply known and accepted just as he or she is.

- Level one: Peak communication—Mutual complete openness, honesty, respect, and love are required to communicate at this level. An all-encompassing intimacy is shared, often involving sexual relationships. A minority of human interactions take place at this level.

In therapeutic communication with clients, it is important for the nurse to have a clear idea about appropriate boundaries that will facilitate healing. A "boundary" refers to the line between a therapeutic and a personal relationship. A boundary will influence your decision about the appropriateness of certain behavior, such as touching or not touching a client. A psychiatric nurse may limit touching to a handshake, whereas a geronto-logical nurse may use supportive physical touch as an adjunct to verbal communication. The nurse must consider how the behavior will affect the relationship and what it will mean to the client.

The goal of therapeutic communication is the development of a professional relationship that will be the context for meeting the client's health needs. This differs from social relationships in which both parties have a right to expect that their needs will be met. When friends communicate, one may share a problem while the other listens and provides support. At another time, roles reverse. In a professional relationship, there will be no expectation that the nurse will get his or her needs met, therefore it is important that the nurse build a support system of friends and colleagues to meet those needs.

If the nurse crosses over a relationship boundary with the client, the interaction will confuse the client, and the nurse will appear to be asking for more than a nurse–client relationship. In a therapeutic relationship, interaction will take place at levels five, four, and three with an occasional interchange at level two, but never at level one.

New professionals may confuse appropriate boundaries and find themselves making errors in judgment, such as spending more time with one client than others because that client meets their needs in some way. The nurse may also avoid a client and neglect his or her needs because something about the relationship is disturbing or anxiety provoking. When the client feels compelled to put the nurse at ease or meet the nurse's needs, a boundary has been crossed. Clients do not need this added anxiety; they need to relax and trust that the nurse has the client's best interests at heart and can manage the healing interaction free of awkwardness or threats to confidentiality and trust.

■ BELIEFS OF EFFECTIVE HELPERS

A.W. Combs[10] and colleagues at the University of Florida conducted research on the characteristics of effective helpers. In their study, helpers were evaluated for their effectiveness, and the most effective helpers responded to specific questions about their beliefs in six major categories. The results are summarized in Table 2-1.

Professionals will act according to what they believe to be their purpose. The purpose of a therapeutic relationship is to listen carefully so that you will come to know your client and understand his or her health needs from the client's perspective. With this understanding, the nurse can use the nursing process and collaborate with other members of the health care team to promote self-care and the highest level of functioning possible.

Carl Rogers[11] suggests seven key questions that lead to a form of self-examination that will help us evaluate the quality of one's helping skills:

1. Can I behave in some way that will be perceived by the other person as trustworthy, as dependable or consistent in some deep sense? Here congruence is the key factor. Whatever feeling or attitude is being experienced must be matched by an awareness of that attitude, and actions must match feelings.

2. Can I be expressive enough as a person that what I am will be communicated unambiguously? The difficulty here is to be fully aware of who one truly is. Rogers says this: "If I can form a helping relationship to myself—if I can be sensitively aware of and acceptant toward my own feelings—then the likelihood is great that I can form a helping relationship toward another."

3. Can I let myself experience positive attitudes toward this other person—attitudes of warmth, caring, liking, interest, respect? This often engenders the fear that if we allow ourselves to openly express these feelings, the client might misinterpret our intentions, and the therapeutic distance might be blurred. The key here is to remain in our professional identities yet still relate in a caring way to the other person.

4. Can I be strong enough as a person to be separate from the other? This question speaks to avoiding identification. I must be ever aware of my own feelings and express them as mine, totally separate from the feelings I may perceive that the client is experiencing. Likewise, I must be strong in my otherness to avoid becoming depressed when my client is depressed, or fearful in the face of my client's fear, or destroyed by his or her anger.

5. Can I let myself enter fully into the world of my client's feelings and personal meanings and see these as he or she does? The key effort here is to avoid judging the client's perspectives but instead allow empathy to occur. In this way, when the world of the other is more fully experienced, the help that is offered can be based on this holistic level of knowing

made possible by empathy. Meanings can be confronted with acceptance and modified to work toward healing. Judgment and criticism of meanings places a barrier between the helper and the client.

6. Can I act with sufficient sensitivity that my behavior will not be perceived as a threat in the relationship? A client who feels free of external fear or threat feels free to examine behavior and change it. Client care is threatening in and of itself. Whatever we can do to lower anxiety will assist the effectiveness of our helping.

7. Can I meet this other individual as a person who is in the process of becoming, or will I be bound by his or her past and by my past? Martin Buber uses the phrase "confirming the other" (transcription of personal communication with C. Rogers, April 18, 1957). This means accepting the whole potentiality of the other—the person he or she was created to become. People will act the way we relate to them. The Pygmalion effect was described following the famous Broadway play in which a poor working girl showed that she could behave like a princess when she was treated like one and taught carefully.

Table 2-1   Summary of the Beliefs of "Effective" Helpers

Combs and associates describe commonly held beliefs and perceptions of effective helpers in six categories:

1. Subject or discipline—One is committed to knowing one's discipline well, and knowledge about one's discipline is so personally integrated and meaningful as to have the quality of beliefs. Effective helpers are committed to discovering the personal meaning of knowledge and converting it to beliefs.

2. Helper's frame of reference—Effective helpers tend to favor an internal frame of reference emphasizing the importance of people's attitudes, feelings, and values that are uniquely human over an external frame of reference that emphasizes facts, things, organization, money, etc.

3. Beliefs about people—Effective helpers believe that people are essentially:
   - Able to understand and deal with their own problems given sufficient time and information
   - Basically friendly and well-intentioned
   - Worthy and have great value; they possess dignity and integrity that must be maintained
   - Essentially internally motivated, maturing from within and striving to grow and help themselves
   - A source of satisfaction in professional work rather than a source of suspicion and frustration

4. Helper's self-concept—Effective helpers have a clear sense of self before they enter into relationships with others. They feel basically fulfilled and adequate, so self-discipline is well practiced. Therapeutic presence for the other is made possible by a strong sense of self, personal fulfillment, and personal adequacy.

5. Helper's purposes—Effective helpers believe that their purpose is to facilitate and assist rather than control people. Their purpose includes honesty, acknowledging personal inadequacies, and need for growth. Another purpose is to be involved and committed to the helping process. They are committed to working out solutions rather than working toward preconceived goals or notions.

6. Beliefs about appropriate methods or approaches to the task—Effective helpers are more oriented toward people than rules and regulations. They are more concerned about people's perceptions than with the objective framework within which they practice. In helping people, the most effective approach is to discover how the world seems to that person. Self-concept is at the heart of the way one views the world, so working with self-concept is imperative. Helpers have to be committed to gaining the trust of clients so that self-control can be relearned in a positive way. The helping relationship makes this growth possible.

Source: Reprinted with permission from Combs, A.W. (1969). *Florida Studies in the Helping Professions.* Gainesville, FL: University of Florida Press.

FACILITATING EMOTIONAL EXPRESSION

Nurses are often present during clients' emotionally charged life experiences including trauma, serious illness, birth, and death. During these times, clients will express a variety of powerful emotions from joy to great distress. Whereas sharing a client's joy brings pleasure, negative emotions may be difficult for the nurse to bear. Nurses who are unprepared for clients' distress may distance themselves by minimizing contact with the distressed client, avoiding conversation, offering false reassurance (e.g., "You will be okay") or changing the subject. Other ways that nurses avoid sharing the client's experience is by talking too much, talking about self, or talking about superficial topics.

Overlooking opportunities to assist clients to express their feelings may result in missed opportunities for client growth. Expression can decrease the negative impact of difficult life situations, lead to greater self-understanding, and promote effective coping. In studies of writing and talking about feelings associated with traumatic events, Pennebaker and associates found that expression of feelings of distress was associated with better physical and emotional outcomes.[12,13] Using empathy, the nurse can notice clients' readiness to express distress, demonstrate willingness to be supportive, and accept the clients' expressions. For best results, the nurse needs to promote the client's rational discussion of experiences, expression of emotions associated with the experience, and self-examination for insights and opportunities for growth.[14]

CONCLUSION

The more a nurse fully comprehends the importance of the nature of helping, the more the nurse will become committed to the growth required for consistent therapeutic use of self. Practice and study are necessary for improvement. Discussing confusing interactions with a mentor or experienced colleague can be very helpful in preventing errors in judgment or at least learning from experience so that they will not be repeated.

REFERENCES

1. Watson, J. (2002). Intentionality and caring-healing consciousness: A practice of transpersonal nursing. *Holistic Nursing Practice, 16*(2), 12–19.

2. Godkin, J., & Godkin, L. (2004). Caring behaviors among nurses: Fostering a conversation of gestures. *Health Care Management Review, 29*(3), 258–267.

3. Peplau, H.E. (1952). *Interpersonal relations in nursing.* New York: Putnam.

4. Hagerty, B.M., & Patusky, K.L. (2003). Reconceptualizing the nurse–patient relationship. *Journal of Nursing Scholarship, 35*(2), 145–150.

5. Davis, C.M. (2006). *Patient practitioner interaction.* Thorofare, NJ: Slack.

6. Davis, C.M. (1982). *A phenomenological description of empathy as it occurs within physical therapists for their clients.* Unpublished doctoral dissertation, Boston University.

7. Stein, E. (1970). *On the problem of empathy* (2nd ed.). The Hague, Netherlands: Martinus Nijhoff.

8. Goleman, D. (1995). *Emotional intelligence.* New York: Bantam Books.

9. Powell, J. (1969). *Why am I afraid to tell you who I am?* Niles, IL: Argus Communications.

10. Combs, A.W., Avila, D.L., & Purkey, W.W. (1971). *Helping relationships—Basic concepts for the health professions* (2nd ed.). Boston: Allyn and Bacon.

11. Rogers, C.R. (1961). The characteristics of a helping relationship. In C. Rogers (Ed.), *On becoming a person.* Boston: Houghton Mifflin.

12. Pennebaker, J.W., & Seagal, J.D. (1999). Forming a story: The health benefits of narrative. *Journal of Clinical Psychology, 55,* 1243–1254.

13. Pennebaker, J.W. (1990). *Opening up: The healing power of confiding in others.* New York: Morrow.

14. Kennedy-Moore, E., & Watson, J. (2001). How and when does emotional expression help? *Review of General Psychology, 5*(3), 187–212.

EXERCISES

1. Communication Style

A. What I like most about the way I communicate with others is . . .

B. I am most comfortable communicating when . . .

C. I am most uncomfortable communicating when . . .

D. What I want to change about the way I communicate with others is . . .

E. I don't know how to say . . .

F. When I want to express my thoughts to loved ones, I usually . . .

G. When I want to communicate my feelings to loved ones, I usually . . .

H. When I have to communicate upsetting information, I usually . . .

Discussion

After you have answered these questions, write a summary of your communication style. In what ways will your communication style affect your relationships with colleagues? With clients?

2. Responding to Situations

Below are situations in which you might find yourself as you interact with clients in the clinical setting. These situations are posed to help you better understand the process of therapeutic interaction.

A. Your client, Mr. Jefferson, is 70 years old and has several health problems including obesity, diabetes, and hypertension. When you visit him in his home to conduct health teaching, you notice that he doesn't seem interested in what you have to say. When you ask about how he has been managing his diabetes, he changes the subject.

What might you feel in this situation?

What questions could you ask to find out what health issues are important to him?

What conflicts might exist between his needs and yours?

B. Mrs. Weslan has a long history of severe psychiatric problems. She is hospitalized briefly for stabilization with medications, and you are assigned to develop a therapeutic relationship with her. Her problems seem overwhelming and you wonder where to begin.

What might you be feeling in this situation?

Is there really anything that you can do that will help?

What would be a rewarding outcome in this situation?

What might be one realistic therapeutic goal in this situation?

Discussion

In your self-assessment notebook, summarize what you have learned about yourself in doing these exercises. What kinds of clients might you be interested in working with when you graduate? What factors have influenced your preferences?

Section 2
Interacting with Others

3

The Process of Helping

Christine L. Williams, DNSc, APRN, BC and Carol M. Davis, DPT, EdD, MS, FAPTA

OBJECTIVES

1. To describe the characteristics of a helping interview

2. To portray the qualities of an effective interviewer

3. To emphasize the importance of both thoughts and feelings in communication

4. To emphasize the importance of effective communication in the initial stages of the relationship

5. To examine the risks and rewards of communicating clearly in the presence of intense feelings

Therapeutic interaction requires new skills, but more than that, it requires unlearning old ways of communicating that will not work in a therapeutic relationship. This chapter is devoted to teaching a new way of communicating with the express purpose of developing a healing alliance with clients.

Remember that the client is not simply the person with an illness or injury, but his or her entire family is your client as well. Be aware of the need to include family members in your assessment and planning. Even when the "identified client" wants your help, the cooperation of supportive family members can make the difference between success and failure of the plan of care.

When clients are ill, they often feel afraid and vulnerable. They may be in the midst of a major life crisis such as birth or death. They may be caring for a family member who is dying. Most people resist giving over some control of their lives to strangers. They may not welcome this encounter with a nurse. The underlying theme in this chapter is to help you communicate in ways that foster opportunities for growth or solve problems while respecting and honoring clients during their health care experience.

As nurses, we recognize that the client may feel at a distinct disadvantage. At least from their perspective, we possess the knowledge and skills to manage the situation. Our interest, genuineness, acceptance, and positive regard are critical to establishing a healing relationship. The trust we foster will influence how much information we obtain during the assessment and how much the client benefits from our help.

■ THE HEALTHCARE ENCOUNTER

Without effective communication, we are unable to acquire objective and subjective information to make health care decisions with our clients, and we are unable to utilize the relationship between nurse and client for therapeutic ends. This chapter focuses on sorting out emotion-laden communication to help clients identify and solve their own problems. Sometimes the first encounter with a client is in the home or outpatient clinic. If there is no emergency, the nurse can focus on collecting comprehensive information to better understand the client. In other situations, encounters are brief. (See Table 3-1.) The context of each interaction will affect the extent of the information collected and the nature of the nurse's approach; however, many principles remain constant.

The interview is the first opportunity to convey a professional healing attitude, and it must be learned and practiced to develop skill. Learning therapeutic communication is like learning a new language. At first

Table 3-1   Brief vs Extended Nurse-Client Interactions

Brief	Extended
Postanesthesia care of client in ambulatory surgery center	Care of a client in hospice
Telephone triage of a sick child	Admission of an older adult to long term care

it will feel awkward. You will wonder if your words sound artificial. Gradually, as you practice, it will sound more and more natural. When you see the results in the trust and confidence of your clients, you will be encouraged to keep working at it.

Your words and inner attitude must be in harmony for the interview to be therapeutic. For the best results, the nurse must feel confident, peaceful, at one with his or her self, and genuinely willing to establish a healing relationship. Take a few deep breaths to relax before you begin. Focusing on the client's needs rather than your own feelings of awkwardness will help you to forget your self-consciousness.

Meeting the Client

Your introduction will include the use of your full name and the client's formal name. After the initial introduction, it is appropriate to ask the client what name he or she would like you to use. Many of us have had the experience of having our names mispronounced or shortened in ways that left us feeling vaguely and unnecessarily uncomfortable. Endearments such as "sweetie" or "mamma" are never appropriate. Your nonverbal behavior must convey respect and warmth. Position yourself at eye level rather than standing over the client as he or she lies in bed or sits in a wheelchair. Lean slightly toward the client to convey interest. Maintaining eye contact while staying at an appropriate social distance (4 feet away) is important in beginning a successful relationship.

Active Listening

Active listening is a form of therapeutic listening that helps the client clearly convey what he or she is trying to say. It involves paraphrasing the client's words to clarify whether or not you have caught the client's intended meaning. You must suspend your thoughts and attend exclusively to the nonverbal behavior and the words of the

other person. *This is not easy* and requires practice. Your goal is to understand rather than judge or defend against. For some, it will require great effort to resist responding with a suggestion of what to do or with an argument. One word you will want to avoid at such times is "but."

Active listening is made up of three different processes:[1]

1. Restatement—repeating the words of the client as you heard them.

   Example: "You better call the doctor because I'm leaving this hospital today!"

   Restatement: "You want to go home today?"

   Restatement can be annoying if not timed appropriately. When done well, it assures the client that you have, indeed, heard what he or she is saying. The main purpose of restatement is to help the client continue speaking and should only be used in the *initial phases* of active listening. When you have reassured the client that you heard his or her words, reflection and clarification become more useful responses.

2. Reflection—verbalizing both the content and the implied feelings of the speaker.

   Example: "No one seems to know what's wrong with me. I've had so many tests and no one tells me anything. I've had it!"

   Reflection: "You're tired of all the tests and frustrated because you still don't know what's wrong?"

   The purpose of reflection is to express in words the feelings and attitudes sensed behind the words of the speaker. This aspect of listening indicates you are hearing more than just the words—you are hearing the emotion behind them. Awareness of feelings is critical to identifying the real problem. Notice the client's nonverbal behavior. Does it reinforce what the client is saying? Does it contradict the client's words? Sometimes we guess incorrectly, but this gives the client the chance to clarify for us and for him- or herself exactly what he or she is feeling. When the nurse wants to help the client to examine both thoughts and feelings, clarification is used.

3. Clarification—summarizing or simplifying the client thoughts and feelings and resolving confused verbalizations into clear, concise statements.

Example: "When the doctor told me I needed some tests, I thought I would be out of here in a couple of days. But I've been sitting here all weekend doing nothing and now you're telling me I still need more tests. I can't stay here; I need to get back to work. I'm not sure what I'm supposed to do. I can't afford to just lie around here another day."

Clarification: "You thought you would be discharged by Friday? Now you realize that the tests are going to take longer than you expected and you are worried about missing work?"

These skills take practice, as does resisting the impulse to fix the problem. In this case, the client may begin to feel some relief just because he or she has been heard and may begin to problem solve on his or her own: "I will call my supervisor and explain that I haven't had a chance to talk to the doctor yet. I don't really want to leave if there is something really wrong."

Nonverbal Communication

We communicate more with nonverbal behavior than we do with words. Our nonverbal behavior conveys how we feel regardless of what we say. The nurse's nonverbal communication can either facilitate or hinder the quality of the interview. Key nonverbal elements of a helping interview include use of space (eliminate physical barriers such as a desk between you and the client), time (minimize interruptions), appropriate posture (avoiding rigid posture, slouching, or defiant gestures), voice inflection (appropriate speed and volume; warmth and genuine interest conveyed versus flatness or excessive use of "you knows"), and eliminating distracting body movements (twitching, shaking foot, tapping pencil).

Congruence

Congruence is a term that indicates that the verbal and nonverbal messages match.[2] For example, congruence is present when the nurse admits that he or she is frustrated or irritated rather than denying those feelings. If the nurse denies feelings, nonverbal responses such as muscle tension and facial expression will communicate the feeling to the client anyway and create confusion. Incongruence appears dishonest or "not ringing true." How often have we been caught in incongruence when someone asks for a compliment: "Well, do you like my new haircut or *not?*" "Well yes, it's okay I guess." What was felt was

less than okay but no one likes to appear rude. When a person is congruent, he or she appears to be open, honest, genuine, and authentic. Nonverbal cues and tone of voice are consistent with the words spoken.

Congruence requires self-awareness. Before speaking, you must consider both feelings and thoughts and reconcile conflicts such as wanting to not be hurtful, yet wanting to be honest. A congruent response to the requested compliment might be: "You know, I noticed you had a new haircut, but I really liked it the old way." With this response, the person realizes that you value honesty and are willing to be honest but can avoid being rude. The message "rings true" and you feel better. More important, the person knows you will resist trying to please others and disregarding your own feelings.

Congruence is best conveyed when it is communicated with sensitivity. It should never be used as a rationalization for insensitive and rude honesty.

Communicating Emotions

Many of us are rather unaware of our day-to-day communication style and are surprised when someone misunderstands the message we have tried to convey. It is difficult to come outside of ourselves and notice how we interact with others. Some of us have been given direct feedback by our friends about our communication. Statements such as, "I love the way you listen carefully to what I say and wait until I'm finished before you respond," vs, "I wish you'd hear me out instead of mentally practicing a quick comeback!" give us clear information about how we are doing as we communicate in that moment.

When strong emotions are communicated, the message may be unclear because the client (or nurse) is upset and unable to clearly identify what the heart of the problem is and how to best go about solving it. To be effective, you must be aware of your emotional reactions and avoid the use of emotion-laden communication (even when you feel personally attacked).

Emotion-laden exchanges are cluttered with intense feelings, derogatory remarks, apologies, and so on. To sort out the problem, special listening skills are needed to defuse the emotion and get at the problem. Resist the desire to respond (unhelpfully) to correct the problem right away to get rid of the client's (or your own) anxiety, anger, or conflict. Too often, we respond by giving quick advice or offering a defensive reply. Instead, use active listening skills.

Case example

Mrs. Mendel, an 82-year-old widow, is admitted to a nursing home accompanied by her daughter, Mrs. Garcia. Mrs. Mendel has lived with her daughter for the past 10 years, however, in the past year she has become increasingly confused and disoriented, and her resistance to eating, bathing, and dressing has made it difficult for her daughter to manage. Her illness is diagnosed as dementia. Mrs. Garcia made the reluctant decision to place her mother in a nursing home and was feeling tremendous guilt about it. She had promised her mother that she would always care for her at home.

Mrs. Garcia visited every day and was often present during mealtimes. Although Mrs. Mendel was gaining weight, Mrs. Garcia was critical of her mother's care and especially the quality of the meals. One day she came to the nurses' station and shouted, "The food you are giving my mother is totally unacceptable. You can't expect her to eat that!"

This is an example of an emotion-laden interaction similar to many that take place daily in hospitals and long-term care facilities. If you were the nurse, how would you have responded? What would you have felt? Would you have become defensive? Would you have argued that Mrs. Mendel was showing remarkable signs of improvement now that she was at the nursing home? Would you have shouted, "Nobody speaks to me that way!"

Situations such as placing a loved one in long-term care involve feelings of loss, vulnerability, and fear. Family members must give over control to strangers, often in institutions that seem strange, impersonal, and frightening with cultures very different from their own. At the root of every emotional outburst is a problem. What, exactly, is the problem in this case example, and whose problem is it? Mrs. Garcia would say that the problem is that her mother is not being treated well. Therefore, the nursing home and food are the problems. The nurse might say that the problem is that Mrs. Garcia is feeling helpless about her mother's illness and lashed out in frustration. Both are correct from their own way of seeing the world. If the nurse maintains that he or she is right, it will not solve the problem. To resolve the problem, it is the nurse's responsibility to take the client's view (in this case, Mrs. Garcia, as Mrs. Mendel's closest relative, is the client). The nurse can resolve this uncomfortable situation and at the same time avoid taking blame for the situation by active listening and the use of "I" messages.

Clear Sending—Use of "I" Statements

When an individual feels distressed and wants to communicate to another person that he or she is upset, clear communication is facilitated with "I" messages. "I" messages ("I think" or "I feel," rather than the commonly used editorial "they," or "you," or "everyone") are most effective for resolving problems.[3]

Many people have a tendency to blame when they feel uncomfortable. An example in which the nurse blames the client might be: "*You* keep making suggestive remarks. I'm not going to be able to help you if *you* keep talking that way." In this case, whose problem is it? If I am upset, the problem is mine. The following response using an "I" message is more likely to resolve the problem: "*I'm* feeling very frustrated. *I'm* trying to help you learn about your diabetes and *I'm* feeling uncomfortable with the things you are saying. Let's talk about this."

With "I" messages, the nurse clearly expresses and takes responsibility for his or her frustration.[4] This way, it is up to the other person to respond, hopefully with concern, perhaps even with active listening. Note, however, that use of an "I" statement does not guarantee that the other person will respond in a helpful way. What it does mean is that the nurse's feelings will be expressed appropriately and those feelings will be less likely to disrupt the relationship. If those feelings are not expressed, they may lead to the nurse avoiding this client who is in need of diabetic teaching.

Using "I" statements involves taking a risk. When the nurse speaks in the first person, he or she takes responsibility for feelings rather than ignoring, disclaiming, or minimizing them. It takes reflective thought to decide what the nurse is feeling and how it can be expressed appropriately. Sending "I" messages tells the other person that you believe this problem can be solved with appropriate, clear, respectful discussion.

The nurse can let Mrs. Garcia know that she is a valued member of the health team and that her contributions to her mother's care are essential to her well-being. A response that helps to establish the nurse's desire to work together with Mrs. Garcia might be "I see that you are very upset and I want to help. Let's sit and talk about this. Please tell me what is wrong." With this approach, the nurse may learn that it is not the food at all that is the problem but that Mrs. Garcia is feeling overwhelmed by many events in her life. After allowing her to express her frustration, she and the nurse may decide that bringing in food from home is one small step toward helping Mrs. Garcia to feel less helpless and to be more involved in her mother's care. When the nurse communicates in a helpful manner, he or she resists the need to respond impulsively, to offer quick advice, or to offer a quick solution to a problem. Instead, the nurse strives to clarify the problem and to assist the person in solving it for him- or herself.

Unhelpful Responses

Unhelpful responses are impulsive and do not reflect caring, warmth, respect, compassion, and empathy. Accepting that the other person is doing the best he or she can in the moment and accepting the responsibility to be therapeutic in the midst of a chaotic situation are actions of a mature health professional. Some examples of unhelpful responses are as follows:

- Offering false reassurances. Statements such as, "She'll be fine, she just needs time to adjust" signal the nurse's unwillingness to listen to clients' perceptions of their problems.

- Dismissing concerns. Statements such as, "Oh, it can't be all that bad," or "If you think you have it bad, you should just look around you," may be used by a nurse who is trying to get away as rapidly as possible.

- Offering judgmental responses. There are several types of judgmental responses, such as responses that convey approval or disapproval, either verbally or nonverbally, at an inappropriate moment. One such verbal response is, "You're really planning to take the baby home to a hotel room?" Another response gives advice at a time when it is more important for the client to make his or her own decision, such as, "You need to leave your husband now before things get any worse!" Another response that is stereotypical and not helpful is, "All parents have to make sacrifices."

- Defensiveness. When we feel threatened, we respond defensively. Defensiveness indicates a personalization and refusal to listen carefully to what the client is saying. A response such as, "We are so understaffed. I am trying to take care of your mother's needs but I have eight other residents to take care

of" may be true but does little to solve the daughter's problem.

As you practice viewing the world from the client's perspective you will more than likely receive cooperation from clients. This view places you in the role of advocate and partner rather than that of authority figure or adversary.

What's Your Style?

Your communication style can make a difference.[5] Norton identified several communication styles, including attentive and dominant styles.[6] Which is more like your style of communicating? If you are client-focused in your approach, and if you use empathy and active listening, you are probably using an attentive style. If you are more focused on what you need to obtain from the interaction (e.g., assessment information or compliance with your teaching) you could be using a dominant style. A dominant style is characterized by focusing the conversation on your agenda, talking too much, and interrupting the client's story. Ask your colleagues to tell you what they observe about how you interact with clients. Consider the fact that an attentive style expands communication whereas the dominant style leaves the other person little opportunity to respond. If your goal is to find out what your clients really feel and need, an attentive style will probably get better results.

■ THE HEALTHCARE INTERVIEW: A UNIQUE FORM OF COMMUNICATING

Interviewing is much more than obtaining a client's history. The interview often sets the stage for the care we give. A client may be seeking health information or may be worried or in pain. He or she may feel in need of our help and understanding. Clients hope that we will listen carefully and that we will know something about their concerns.

Helpful Attitudes

Not only is it important to convey an accepting attitude for our clients during the interview, it is imperative that the client feels listened to and understood so that all of the important information can surface that will lead to the most adequate and complete understanding of the client's concern. Thus, effective clinical decision making depends on skillful interviewing.

The Healing Attitude of the Interview

Clients are simply people who need our professional help to identify their health needs and to help them achieve their best possible health state. Nurses who have an attitude that facilitates healing are able to accept their clients just as they are without judging them. These nurses will have identified and dealt with their own biases and prejudices about certain behaviors such as alcohol abuse, smoking, use of profanity, lack of motivation to change, obesity, etc. They will have determined that they are willing to be therapeutic even when the client does not behave as the nurse would. As much as possible, they will be aware of and willing to put aside prejudices about culture and ethnicity, gender, age, or sexual orientation. As much as we might dislike a client's behavior, it is helpful to believe that the client would have acted differently if he or she had more information and had been less impulsive.

Alfred Benjamin[7] says:

When interviewing, we are left with what we are. We have no books then, no classroom lessons, and no supporting person at our elbow. We are alone with the individual who has come to seek our help. How can we assist him (or her)? The same basic issues will confront us afresh whenever we face an interviewee for the first time. In summary they are:

1. Shall we allow ourselves to emerge as genuine human beings, or shall we hide behind our role, position, and authority?

2. Shall we really try to listen with all our senses to the interviewee?

3. Shall we try to understand him (her) with empathy and acceptance?

4. Shall we interpret his (her) behavior to him (her) in terms of his (her) frame of reference, our own, or society's?

5. Shall we evaluate his (her) thoughts, feelings, and actions, and if so, in terms of whose values: his (hers), society's, or ours?

6. Shall we support, encourage, urge him (her) on so that by leaning on us hopefully he (she) may be able to rely on his (her) own strength one day?

7. Shall we question and probe, push and prod, causing him (her) to feel that we are in command and that once all our queries have been answered, we shall provide the solutions he (she) is seeking?

8. Shall we guide him (her) in the direction we feel certain is the best for him (her)?

9. Shall we reject his (her)… thoughts and feelings, and insist that he (she) become like us, or at least conform to our perception of what he (she) should become?

These are the central attitudinal questions that underlie every helping interview. When you read the above questions carefully, you will see that Benjamin phrases a few to encourage a negative response, as if to have us examine our attitudes very carefully to be clear about our helping intentions. When a healing attitude is established, skillful and artful questions will follow, and the interview will become one more important tool in the nurse's repertoire of healing behaviors. When this routine becomes second nature, less stress will be attached to it and you will experience great pleasure listening to most of your clients tell their story.

The Interview

Timing

With regard to timing, an effective interviewer avoids interrupting (which often reveals an underlying harmful attitude of "this person is not very important to me") and listens carefully using silence. Nurses who are uncomfortable with silence will miss much of what a person says if the client were given a chance to pause and reflect. A specific amount of time is set to spend listening to the client as he or she tells you his or her story. The amount of time will vary with the situation. Generally, less time is available in an emergency and more time is allotted when the client's need is less urgent (e.g., admission to long-term care, ambulatory settings when the focus is health promotion or preventative care).

> Sally H. came to the emergency room complaining of abdominal pain. The nurse used an attentive communication style and listened while Sally told her "story" in her own way. By using active listening skills, the nurse discovered that Sally's actual reason for coming was that she had been raped.

Listening to the client's "story" will give you the most accurate accounting of the reason for seeking help.

The information you obtain from the client will not always follow the structured format that is found on a data collection form, but by allowing the client to explain the situation in his or her own way, the most important information will have a chance to surface in the conversation. The nurse can fill in the gaps later. If the client is highly anxious, he or she will need the nurse's guidance to explain fully. Guidance should be kept to a minimum to determine what the client believes is important and what he or she is seeking in this encounter. General information is obtained first, allowing the client to become comfortable and to begin in his or her own way. More specific requests for information, especially sensitive information, can be obtained later after rapport has developed.

Stages of the Interview

There are four stages in the interview: the preparation phase, orientation phase, working phase, and termination phase.

Probably the most difficult part of communicating with clients is getting started. Students often delay meeting their clients to read health records or obtain information from other nurses. Although these activities have value, there is no substitute for communicating directly with the client. Anticipation of the encounter can lead to a number of concerns, such as will the client like me? Will he or she refuse to talk to me? What should I do if the client's family is visiting or if the client is talking on the phone?

Preparation Phase

The preparation phase takes place before meeting the client. Clinical supervision is an important part of the preparation process and is used as an ongoing method of helping to improve therapeutic communication skills. It is critical to meet with a faculty member or, for the practicing nurse, an experienced clinician to discuss any concerns about meeting with the client and how to proceed. Guidance from a more experienced person is considered to be an integral part of professional practice. Through the relationship with a supervisor, the student or nurse learns more about the therapeutic use of self. The supervisor can assist the nurse to examine his or her feelings about the client.

To assist in the process of supervision, the interview may be audiotaped or videotaped. This allows an accurate review and critique of the interaction. When taping is impossible due to institutional policies, process recording can be substituted. In process recording, the student or nurse writes the conversation verbatim from memory immediately following the interview. The written version is shared with the supervisor and discussed. Although this process is not as accurate as recording an interview as it happens, it is a useful learning tool.

Kotecki[8] identified a process called *affirming the self* that was used by student nurses to prepare for communicating with clients. Affirming the self consists of using techniques such as positive self-talk to improve their readiness to engage in a new relationship with clients. Each of us engages in an inner dialogue continuously as we go about our daily activities. This dialogue can be self-critical, leading to increased anxiety and discomfort. For example, when students report self-talk such as, "This patient will be hard to talk to," or, "I know I am going to make a fool of myself," their likely response will be anxiety. Under these circumstances, no wonder the student avoids the encounter! When self-talk is positive and supportive, students approach a new situation with confidence, for example, "I know I can handle this situation. I've been successful before, I can do it again." When we find ourselves engaging in negative self-talk, we can tell ourselves to "Stop!" and redirect our thoughts to a more positive theme.

Consider the environment you have chosen for the interview to be sure it is as comfortable as possible. Temperature, lighting, and seating arrangements are examples of factors that can influence how much the client is willing to talk. In the hospital or home, the nurse needs to have comfortable seating as well as the client. If the nurse is standing, this sends a message "I am not staying long." The client's inner state is important as well. The client is not likely to communicate freely if he or she is in pain or suffers other physical discomforts. Take the time to provide comfort first.

Your demeanor will also influence the client's reaction to the encounter. Is your manner of dress that of a competent professional? Your self-esteem is reflected in the care you take with your appearance. Your style of dress communicates messages about how you view your role as a nurse. The client will be more likely to develop trust in an individual who is self-assured and professional in appearance. Identification badges are important as well. When the client can read your name and title, he or she can be assured of who you are and what he or she can expect.

Orientation Phase

The orientation phase of the interview takes place as you, the interviewer, meet the client and explain who you are, why you are here, and the purpose of the interview and the amount of time you will spend with the client. Termination of the relationship begins at this initial step as you clarify what to expect. Be as clear as you can about how long this interview will last and whether future sessions are anticipated. It is important to provide as much privacy as possible at the first meeting so the client will be comfortable about bringing up his or her concerns. Although you may feel rushed, communicate patience and attentiveness to be effective. On a busy morning, you may have only 5 minutes to spend with a client, but you can give the client your undivided attention for those 5 minutes and arrange to come back later to continue the interview.

Establishing rapport is facilitated by beginning with a brief social exchange. This type of communication is called the "ice breaker." It is a way of making the client comfortable before the business of the interview begins. Whether you are visiting a client in a healthcare setting or in his or her home, you can use the environment to get clues about how to begin. Asking about a greeting card or family photograph displayed on a bedside table is one example of an "ice breaker." The client may have been engaged in an activity, such as a hobby, just before you arrived. By asking about the activity, you show your interest in the client as a person rather than simply a healthcare "problem."

Working Phase

The body of the interview is the working phase. In this stage, rapport has been developed and the client begins to discuss his or her health issues. A good interviewer will guide the client, assisting the client to explore his or her situation, but not allowing the conversation to drift from the focus of the interaction. Active listening helps the client to clarify the unique aspects of his or her story. The interviewer listens carefully and sorts the information, jotting down significant revelations as he or she prepares for the clinical examination. The body of the interview unfolds in a unique story that the client is encouraged to tell. The helpful interviewer communicates to the client that he or she is being heard by a skilled and caring nurse. When moving from one topic to another, it is helpful to use a transition statement. An example would be: "I think I understand about your headaches; I'd like to hear about your sleep patterns now."

Termination Phase

The termination phase of the interview takes place at a time that has been predetermined by the interviewer. If it becomes obvious that the interview is not complete, the interviewer does not just let the session drop but says, for example, "We're beginning to run out of time for this session and I realize you haven't yet finished. What needs to be covered yet?" Then a second session is scheduled. It is advisable to complete the discussion of the problem before beginning the physical examination. As an interviewer you will be dividing your attention if you try to obtain meaningful information while engaging in palpation and physical evaluation methods. Further, the client will feel vulnerable and exposed and is less likely to share information.

In an ongoing relationship with a client, there may be several meetings over a period of time. When the time of termination is known, it is the nurse's responsibility to give adequate preparation so that termination does not come as a surprise. The client already knows approximately when the relationship will end because you provided the information during the orientation phase. Reminders about termination should come at the beginning of any session rather than at the end to give the client adequate opportunity to discuss it. The client needs an opportunity to discuss what has been gained and to express any unmet needs. The nurse can then make referrals for additional health care if needed.

Sometimes clients resist ending an interview. Establishing trust involves telling the client what to expect and following through on what you have promised. If a home visit is scheduled to be one hour, for example, it is best to leave as scheduled rather than be persuaded to stay longer without any clear purpose. If important concerns prolong the visit, discuss the change and renegotiate the time frame for the visit. Sometimes the client seems to be prolonging the session unnecessarily. In this case, congruence is conveyed by stating that you are leaving and then walking in the direction of the door, as opposed to stating that you are leaving but remaining seated as the client continues to talk.

Body of the Interview: Gathering Information

The key information that is obtained in the interview includes the following:

1. What is the reason for this healthcare encounter?

2. What is the client's perception of the problem?

3. What does the client expect from this interaction? What does he or she hope that you will do?

4. What is the exact nature of the healthcare concern?

5. What are the characteristics of the situation? When did it begin? Precipitating factors? What alleviates the problem? What make it worse? What factors are associated with it?

These are central questions that arise in most healthcare interviews. When you become comfortable with interviewing, you will get the answers without dominating the conversation. You will also notice that you are less stressed in the process, and listening to the client's story is generally a pleasurable, rewarding experience.

■ CONCLUSION

If you have ever been fortunate enough to have observed an experienced nurse at work, you have seen a person who truly values the interview and devotes the kind of attention to it described in this chapter. The greatest obstacles to consistent use of the helping interview are overwork and burnout. The more we feel overextended in our day and the more we feel that we are repeatedly facing irresolvable problems, the more difficult it will be to come outside of ourselves with a therapeutic presence during the interview. The very foundation of the helping interview is a commitment to keeping a balance in our lives so that we are rested and have the energy to give to our work. We have a right to keep a reasonable pace. It is our responsibility to make sure we have as much of ourselves to give as we can.

REFERENCES

1. Munson, P.J., & Johnson, R.B. (1972). *Humanizing instruction or helping your students up the staircase.* Chapel Hill, NC: Johnson Self Instructional Package.

2. Rogers, C.R. (1967). *The therapeutic relationship and its impact.* Madison, WI: University of Wisconsin Press.

3. Davis, C.M. (2006). *Patient practitioner interaction.* Thorofare, NJ: Slack.

4. Grover, S.M. (2005). Shaping effective communication skills and therapeutic relationships at work. *AAOHN Journal, 53*(4), 177–182.

5. Coeling, H.V., & Cukr, P.L. (2000). Communication styles that promote perceptions of collaboration, quality, and nurse satisfaction. *Journal of Nursing Care Quality, 14*(2), 63–74.

6. Norton, R.W. (1978). Foundation of a communicator style construct. *Human Communication Research, 4,* 99–112.

7. Benjamin, A. (1987). *The helping interview* (2nd ed.). Boston: Houghton Mifflin.

8. Kotecki, C.N. (2002). Baccalaureate nursing students' communication process in the clinical setting. *Journal of Nursing Education, 41*(2), 61–68.

EXERCISES

1. Becoming a Professional Helper

In your self-assessment notebook, respond to each of the following questions:

I first became aware that I wanted to help others when . . .

I feel good when I know I have helped another because . . .

I prefer helping people who . . .

When someone refuses my help, I feel . . .

When someone does not seem to help him- or herself, I feel . . .

Discussion

After answering each of the above questions, summarize the major reasons that you decided to make helping others your life's work. What is rewarding about helping others? What frustrations may occur in helping others? How will you achieve a balance between helping and encouraging self-reliance?

2. Responding to Situations

Below are situations in which you might find yourself as you interact with clients in the clinical setting. These situations are posed to help you explore what you might feel and say in the situation.

A. You are scheduled to interview Mr. Reynolds in his home and report your findings to your clinical instructor. There has been a misunderstanding about the time of your visit, and Mr. Reynolds has been waiting for you for over an hour, pacing up and down. When you go to introduce yourself to him, he turns to you angrily and says, "You don't give a damn about other people's time. Don't you realize how long I've been waiting?"

How might you feel at this moment?

What feelings do you think the client is experiencing?

What are some specific things you might say or do at this point to try to demonstrate empathy?

B. You walk into a client's room, and he is watching television. You introduce yourself, and the patient never even takes his eyes off the TV. He acts as if you are not present in the room. How might you feel?

What might be the client's situation?

What self-talk strategies might you use to manage your discomfort in this situation?

C. You are completing an initial assessment on a child who has been admitted to the hospital. The child and her mother are homeless, and the child has an acute upper respiratory infection. The child's clothes are old and dirty, and it appears that she has not been bathed in a long time.

What might you feel?

What approaches to communicating would be helpful? Not helpful?

D. You are trying to conduct an interview with an 85-year-old client, but each time you ask her a question, her adult daughter answers it for her.

What might you feel?

What might be underlying this situation?

What are some things you might say or do to get more information from the client herself?

E. You are interviewing a client and he suddenly leans forward, grabs your arm and says, "You are so attractive. Are you married?"

How might you feel?

What might be underlying the client's behavior?

What might you say or do to get the interview back on track?

Discussion

In your self-assessment notebook, summarize what you have learned about yourself in completing these exercises. Which of the above situations would be most challenging for you? Are there other situations that you can think of that might be uncomfortable for you? Write about a client situation different from those listed above that would be awkward or uncomfortable. Write about what you would feel and how you might respond appropriately.

3. Active Listening

Active listening involves restatement (of the words of the sender), reflection (of the words and underlying feelings of the sender), and clarification (summarizes and focuses the sender's message). Practice writing all three types of responses as requested below.

Restatement

Client	Response from You
I'm very worried about my husband's blood sugar. It seems to be very high most days.	You're worried about your husband's blood sugar being so high.
I used to be able to walk up a flight of stairs without stopping, but now I can only climb one or two steps.	
The nurse practitioner told me about several treatment options to consider. I just don't know what to do.	

Reflection

Client	Response from You
This pain has been going on for months now. I just wish someone would fix it for me.	Your pain just drags on and you wish to relieve it. Perhaps you're concerned that it will never go away?
Yesterday was a good day, but today I feel the same old way.	
It's hard remembering to do my exercises. I want to get better, but it's hard.	

Clarification

Client	Response from You
I wish someone would tell me what's going on with my knees. When I get up in the morning they're fine, but by noon they're swollen and feel tired. I'm too young to be suffering with joint problems. Is this arthritis or what? Do I have to live with this forever?	You're worried that your knee problem might be arthritis and that you'll never be rid of it?
When they told me my son had learning problems I just didn't know what to think. I don't believe in giving a child mind-altering pills, but his teachers say he is failing at school. I don't know how to help him.	
I almost didn't make it here. I got a horrible headache as I was driving here. The traffic is so stressful in this city. Will it ever end? New cars every day on the road. I don't know if I can keep up driving with these headaches. Is there anything you can do for me?	

4

Communication Strategies

Christine L. Williams, DNSc, APRN, BC

OBJECTIVES

1. To compare different types of questions used in communicating with clients

2. To analyze when to use open- and closed-ended questions

3. To describe a progression of questioning

4. To discuss therapeutic communication strategies

5. To analyze barriers to therapeutic communication

6. To delineate guidelines for conveying upsetting information

▪ LEARNING NEW COMMUNICATION SKILLS

Fear of not knowing what to say is a common concern voiced by many students[1] and nurses alike. Nurses sometimes worry that they will not know what to say or will say the wrong thing. This is a normal part of being uncomfortable in an unfamiliar situation. These worries arise when the nurse is focusing on him- or herself rather than the client. These fears will lessen when the nurse focuses on what the client is experiencing in the situation. When the nurse is using empathy, it is more difficult to be self-conscious and awkward.

The art and science of nursing depends upon skillful communication. The experienced nurse brings together a healthy sense of self, empathy and compassion, knowledge of the interview format, and constructive strategies for obtaining and conveying information. Everything we do or say communicates some kind of message. Therefore, it is important to master specific strategies that will facilitate the therapeutic relationship. In this chapter, guidelines for communicating in ways that are helpful will be presented.

▪ QUESTIONING

Sometimes clients talk continuously with very little encouragement from the nurse. Other clients are very reluctant to share information and questioning becomes important in obtaining information. When the information the client offers is not sufficient for understanding health needs, skillful questioning can be used to obtain the missing information. There are many kinds of questions that can be used to obtain information, and some are more useful in therapeutic interactions.

Some questions are more threatening than others and must be reserved until rapport has been developed. Asking about a client's feelings too early in the interaction can be perceived as threatening. This kind of questioning may result in the client becoming defensive or denying emotions. It can be difficult to face emotions and admit them to another person, especially a stranger. Therefore, it is best to wait until the client has developed a degree of comfort in talking with you about his or her situation before you ask him or her to share feelings.

Progression of Questions

When meeting the client for the first time, the nurse guides the client to tell his or her complete "story." This includes an explanation of what has been happening in the client's life and what has happened that led to this encounter with the nurse. Certain types of questions are useful in getting the conversation started while others are more helpful after rapport has been developed.

The healthcare encounter begins with *broad openings,* such as "Tell me about yourself" or "Tell me about your family." Broad openings are designed to give the client the freedom to tell his or her story in whatever way is most comfortable. Often, clients skip over details that are important to the nurse; therefore, it is important to ask questions that will facilitate descriptions of events over time.

Questions That Elicit Description

Questions designed to obtain descriptions are used next. Descriptive questions include those that begin with "Who?" "What?" "Where?" and "When?" When the reason for the healthcare encounter is illness or an accident, it is important to find out how it all began. Ask what happened or when the symptoms began. Descriptive questions can help the nurse to obtain a visual picture of the circumstances of an event, such as a seizure. Ask the client to describe where and when the event took place, who was there, what was said, and to place events in time sequence. This critical information should be documented with key statements quoted directly. It is the professional nurse's responsibility to conduct an initial assessment when a client is admitted to the health care system. Such specific information is useful for other members of the health care team and can prevent their asking the same sensitive questions over and over.

Open-Ended and Closed-Ended Questions

Questions that are *open-ended* are worded to encourage the client to give explanations or to elaborate on a topic. These questions cannot be answered with one or two words. "What happened yesterday?" is an example of an open-ended question. Whenever possible, begin the conversation with open-ended questions. Open-ended questions are also useful later in the interaction to help the client express his or her feelings. "What is it like for you taking care of a sick child for so long?" Open-ended questions are extremely valuable in developing a therapeutic relationship. They provide direction and keep the conversation focused on health care concerns while al-

lowing clients the opportunity to express their concerns in their own words. If the student practices asking open-ended questions when meeting a new client, he or she will often be surprised at how quickly rapport develops.

Closed-ended questions are worded in such a way that they can be answered in one or two words. Many times the nurse needs a specific piece of information, and the closed-ended question is the most efficient way to obtain that information. For example, eventually in every admission interview the nurse asks, "Are you allergic to any medications?" Other examples of closed-ended questions include, "What is today's date?" or "Are you in pain?" Although closed-ended questions are necessary at times, they can prevent the development of a smooth flow of conversation. It is best to avoid them at the beginning of a conversation unless a specific piece of information is needed urgently, such as "Did you take any insulin today?"

When nurses or student nurses are anxious, they are more likely to ask the client closed-ended questions one after another. This limits the flow of conversation to short answers and may lead to inferring that the client does not want to talk. If this happens, reflect on the format of your questions and switch to asking open-ended questions.

General and Specific Questions

In some cases, clients have difficulty answering questions. The nurse may be interested in obtaining descriptions of the client's pain experience and begins the assessment with an open-ended question. "Tell me about your pain" may lead to no response or a limited response, such as "I don't know." It is always best to obtain information in the client's own words, but if the client is unable to explain, it may be necessary to provide some guidance. In these situations, the nurse progresses to more specific questions, such as a closed-ended question: "Does it hurt when I press here?" Another type of question that limits the client's response is the *forced-choice* question. The client must choose between two alternatives. Examples include, "Is your pain sharp or dull?" "Do you feel it more here or there?" Although useful, these questions do not encourage the client to answer with a more accurate alternative. Finally, the *laundry-list* question provides a series of choices: "Do you feel annoyed, frustrated, or angry?" These questions are less valuable because the client must choose from the list provided rather than putting the feeling into his or her own words. In some situations, such as clients with limited ability to speak, these questions may be effective in obtaining some response when the open-ended question leads only to silence.

Questions about Thoughts

After the basic facts are obtained, the nurse encourages the client to describe his or her thoughts about the information. Each client has his or her own unique way of interpreting events, and these evaluations will influence the client's response to the events. With information about the client's thoughts, the nurse will uncover misinterpretations and misinformation that can be addressed in health teaching at a later time. For example, Mrs. Bouchard describes extreme conflict with her adolescent daughter over breaking a curfew. The nurse asks, "What did you think when your daughter did not come home on time?" Mrs. Bouchard replies that her daughter must not care about her parents very much because if she did she would not cause them to worry. The mother's conclusions about the meaning of her daughter's behavior caused an emotional response of hurt and anger that was not helpful to resolving the problem. The nurse also notes that the client will need teaching about adolescence and the issues related to that stage of development.

Questions about Feelings

When the client's thoughts are clarified, it is helpful to encourage recognition of the feelings associated with the situation. Recognizing feelings and expressing them appropriately will bring a feeling of relief and will allow the client to better understand what he or she is experiencing. Feelings can be frightening, and many people are accustomed to ignoring or denying their feelings. The nurse's goal is to give the client permission to share feelings rather than to place demands on him or her when he or she may not be ready to express emotions. One of the most common emotions observed in clinical settings is sadness and grief.

If a client appears sad or ready to cry, the nurse can comment in a supportive tone of voice: "You look very sad right now." This sharing of the nurse's observations serves to bring the emotion to the client's attention. The supportive message suggests to the client that the nurse is willing to share the painful feelings. This often results in the client becoming tearful. It is important that the nurse stay with the client until the crying has ended without

trying to prevent expression of the feelings. Being present for someone who is crying can be uncomfortable. The nurse may have the urge to tell the client to stop crying or to give false reassurances such as, "Everything will work out for the best." This has the effect of closing off the expression of emotions. The message is, "I do not wish to be burdened with your painful feelings." Be aware of your nonverbal behavior. If you hand the client a tissue you may communicate that it is time to stop crying and dry your tears. A hug or even a touch on the client's hand can interrupt the expression of emotion. Wait until clients finish expressing sadness to console them.

In every new situation, clients will experience some degree of anxiety.[2] The tension that results from anxiety will be expressed in behavior such as restlessness or talkativeness. Helping the client to recognize and understand their anxiety will be comforting in itself. Comments such as, "I notice that you are restless" or "Many people are a bit nervous when they come to the hospital," may help clients pinpoint their own anxiety. If the client believes that being anxious is a sign of weakness, he or she will tend to deny it when asked. When the nurse conveys that it is acceptable to be anxious, a direct question will often be helpful. Asking "Are you feeling nervous right now?" may then be answered with a "Yes!" This admission of anxiety makes it possible to offer help with relaxation strategies.

Helping the client to express other basic emotions, such as sadness or anger, requires observation on the part of the nurse. The nurse observes for evidence of emotional responses in the client. Clients can be feeling a strong emotion but can be unaware of that emotion at a conscious level. If the nurse confronts the client when he or she is unaware of the feeling, the client may simply deny it. This is frustrating for the nurse, and it is not helpful for the client. For example, the nurse observed that Mrs. Bouchard seemed angry. Her facial muscles were tense and her fists were clenched during the description of her daughter's behavior. The nurse asked, "What are you feeling right now?" Mrs. Bouchard answered, "I don't know. I thought we would always be so close, like good friends." When asked about what she was feeling directly, she was unable to put it into words. She told the nurse her thoughts rather than her feelings. To help Mrs. Bouchard express her feelings, the nurse commented about her nonverbal behavior. "I notice that you are clenching your fists when you speak about your daughter. Could it be that you are angry?"

Emotional expression is part of communication, and sharing feelings is a very important supportive function of the nurse. Students sometimes worry that they "caused" the feeling. A comment such as, "I made my client cry!" expresses this concern. When clients are sad about the losses they experience, tears may be unexpressed until a supportive person is available to share them. A student who makes him- or herself available may have the privilege of sharing in this powerful human experience.

"Why?" Questions

Asking why may seem to be a simple way to gain an understanding of a client's problems, but "why?" is actually very difficult to answer truthfully. Questions that begin with why are confrontational and often put the client on the defensive. With a why question, you are asking the client to do something that is at the least uncomfortable and may even be impossible, which is to explain or defend his or her actions or beliefs. Such a question can interfere with the development of a therapeutic relationship and is never considered therapeutic.

Multiple Questions

Ask only one question at a time. Although this seems obvious, nurses and nursing students often ask two or more questions without pausing for an answer. Under these conditions, the client may react with anxiety and be less likely to respond at all. At best, he or she can only answer one question at a time. In the following example, the client will be more likely to avoid answering a question about emotions and answer the second, less threatening question instead.

> Nurse: "Are you feeling sad? Would you like to call your husband?"
>
> Client: "No, that's okay."

■ SILENCE

Sometimes words are not necessary and silence can express support. Silence is very effective in facilitating communication when the client is having difficulty expressing his or her thoughts. The nurse's willingness to wait quietly demonstrates patience and acceptance. Silence is also effective when the client is struggling to express feelings. Nurses are often surprised at how grateful clients feel when the nurse remains with them in silence while they express strong emotions.

The use of silence is uncommon in every day social interactions and may take practice before the nurse becomes comfortable with it. It may feel like you are not "doing enough" while staying quietly with a client. Time may seem to pass slowly. Becoming comfortable with the use of silence may be difficult, but the rewards are great.

Table 4-1   Communication Techniques: Therapeutic Strategies

Therapeutic Strategy	Definition	Example
Sharing observations	The nurse shares his or her perceptions with the client	"I notice that you are very talkative today."
General leads	Encouraging the client to continue speaking	"Go on" "Uh-huh" "Okay"
Identifying themes	The nurse shares consistent topics or issues that arise in the client's conversation	"I notice that your disappointment about your son keeps coming up."
Focusing	Asking the client to elaborate on a specific topic	"I would like to hear more about your sleep difficulties."
Voicing doubt	Expressing gentle disbelief to avoid reinforcing the client's misperceptions	The client tells the nurse that her daughter doesn't care about her feelings. The nurse responds, "Really?"
Presenting reality	The nurse presents his or her view of reality	"I know you think the staff is trying to poison you, but I don't believe that is true."

■ COMMUNICATION STRATEGIES

Certain techniques that foster or facilitate communication can be learned (Table 4-1). When these techniques are used within the guidelines discussed previously, they can be helpful in the development of a therapeutic relationship.

Barriers to Communication

A common barrier to communication is a client's limited use of the English language. It is not uncommon to provide care to clients whose primary language is not English. The client may converse in social situations in English but be unfamiliar with medical terminology. To be sure you have an accurate health assessment and can communicate important information, such as discharge teaching, an interpreter is necessary.[3] Another issue arises when the nurse's primary language is not English. Speaking to coworkers or others around you in a language that the client does not understand isolates the client and interferes with the therapeutic relationship. In addition, the client may understand a comment that you did not wish to be heard and understood.

The use of jargon is also common in health care settings and can also confuse and isolate the client. Turning to a group of colleagues to discuss the client's situation in technical terms undermines the client's ability to participate in the interaction and demonstrates a lack of regard for his or her dignity and autonomy.

Avoid sounding "all knowing," such as saying, "I know just how you feel." These false statements do not reassure the client and lead to mistrust since they are obviously not truthful. They convey the message that you do not have to listen because you already know. Addi-

tional examples of nontherapeutic communication are offered in Table 4-2.

■ SELF-DISCLOSURE

Nurses have been socialized to avoid intimacy and to value emotional control and detachment. These attitudes may date back to Florence Nightingale, stoicism and British culture, or the need to professionalize nursing.[4] Sharing some thoughts and feelings with clients has been found to be beneficial in promoting therapeutic conversations with older adults with dementia.[5] How much self-disclosure is helpful? When is it harmful? Obviously, we are not helpful if we burden our clients with our problems. If you are doing most of the talking, you are talking too much. If the conversation focuses on you and your concerns, you are disclosing too much. Sharing your thoughts has the potential for benefit if you share just enough to let the client know that you understand and want to help.

> **Client:** I have to decide whether to tell them to turn off my mother's ventilator. She is 89 years old, and I think that is what she would want. We never talked about it, but I think it is cruel to keep her on machines, don't you?
>
> **Nurse:** I agree with you, I think it is best in this situation.

In this example, the nurse shares her opinion with the client. It may be comforting to the client to know that the nurse agrees, but the nurse's comment also implies approval. When you begin to approve and disapprove of the client's thoughts or behaviors, you create a relationship in which the client knows she or he will be

Table 4-2   Communication Techniques: Nontherapeutic Strategies

Nontherapeutic Strategy	Definition	Example
Giving approval	Judging the client by suggesting that he or she did the "right" thing	"I'm proud of the way you stood up to your husband in the family meeting."
Giving disapproval	Judging the client by suggesting that he or she did the "wrong" thing	"Getting up at noon isn't going to help your depression."
Minimizing	Suggesting the client's experience is unimportant	"I wouldn't worry about it. Everyone goes through that."
Changing the subject	Refusing to follow the client's lead in conversation	"Let's talk about something more pleasant."

judged. Many clients will feel the need to seek the nurse's approval and avoid disapproval. Having to seek a nurse's approval detracts from the client's autonomy and control.

Williams and Irurita[6] studied clients' perceptions of interpersonal interactions with nurses during hospitalization. Interactions that brought a sense of emotional comfort were described by clients who had been hospitalized. Clients perceived a sense of personal control as an important part of emotional comfort. As nurses, we can promote clients' sense of control and thus promote comfort.

In the next example, the nurse shares but does not approve.

With this response, the nurse shares a personal detail but does not burden the client with her own problems or

> Client: I have to decide whether to tell them to turn off my mother's ventilator. She is 89 years old, and I think that is what she would want. We never talked about it, but I think it is cruel to keep her on machines, don't you?
>
> Nurse: Only you can decide. My mother is also 89 years old so I can imagine how difficult this must be for you.

issues. The nurse refrains from giving advice (e.g., "I think you should wait until your brother arrives from out of town.") and from giving approval. This level of sharing is not harmful and may foster a greater sense of support and empathy. Nurses need to be careful that the identification with the client ("My mother is 89 years old and could be in this same situation in the near future") does not lead to over involvement, clouded judgment, or advice giving.

■ DIFFICULT INTERACTIONS WITH CLIENTS

As nurses, we sometimes find ourselves in situations with clients who are uncomfortable. This is the ideal time to seek supervision from a faculty member if you are a student or an experienced clinician if you are a practicing nurse. An objective view can make the difference between a pleasant learning experience and a painful one.

■ CONVEYING UPSETTING INFORMATION

One of the most challenging types of communication for nurses is reporting distressing information to the client. It may be as simple as having to tell the client that

Table 4-3   Difficult Interactions

Situation	Example	Therapeutic Response
Client asks for personal information	"I would like your phone number/home address so that I can keep in touch after I go home."	"I'm sorry but I cannot give my phone number/home address. Are you concerned that you will not be able to reach a team member after you go home?"
	"Do you have children?"	"Yes. Tell me about your family."
Client offers gift	"You have been so good to me. I want you to have this." (offers money)	"I appreciate the thought, but I cannot accept it. I enjoyed getting to know you."
Client asks for a favor	"I haven't been out in so long. Will you pick up a few things for me at the store? I'll give you some money."	"I am here to help you with your health problems. I'd like to understand what happened before you came into the hospital."
Client refuses to talk to you	"Please go away. I don't want to talk."	"I will be available to talk with you from 10:00 to 10:30 today. I will be sitting at the desk right over there. Let me know if you change your mind."

he will not be going home for the weekend although he was looking forward to it with great anticipation. Or it may be that a family member has called to cancel a long-awaited visit. What these situations have in common is that they evoke a feeling of loss. Knowing this in advance will allow the nurse to prepare for expressions of anger and grief. Providing support and allowing the client sufficient time to express the emotions that accompany loss is part of the process on conveying unwelcome information.

Nurses will often be in a position to talk with clients and families in crisis during serious illness, tragic situations, and major life events such as birth and death. What the nurse says and how it is communicated can facilitate acceptance and will often be remembered long after other details of the situation are forgotten. Was the nurse supportive? Caring? Did he or she take time to be with the client and show interest in his or her situation?

How can we communicate frightening, sad, or discouraging information in the most constructive manner possible and encourage questions and further discussion?

Radziewicz and Baile[7] outline a six-step process for communicating in these situations: S-setting, P-perception, I-invitation, K-knowledge, E-emotion, and S-summary.

The *setting* for such important communication should be private and comfortable. Create an atmosphere in which the client will be comfortable expressing emotions. Include individuals whom the client would like to have around for support. It is easier when those involved get the same information at the same time. They can help one another remember and understand what was said. A transition statement such as, "The news is not as good as we had hoped," helps to prepare the client for what is to come.

Perception refers to what the client and supportive others already understand about the situation. Knowing what they already know allows the nurse to uncover misinformation and to build on what they already understand. The nurse may be surprised to find that the client already has at least some knowledge about the situation.

Invitation involves finding out how much the client wants to know at that time or how much information he or she is ready to take in. "Would you like me to explain more about what happened?"

Knowledge is introduced slowly while assessing the client's ability to cope with the information. If an individual is not ready to cope with frightening information,

he or she may use one of several methods to defend against overpowering anxiety. The client may seem to not hear the information, may deny it, or may seem to forget the information soon after it is conveyed. For some, denial may last a few minutes or hours; for others, it may last days or weeks. With time, denial usually gives way to awareness as the client seeks the opportunity to discuss fears with a supportive person. Denial protects the individual from severe discomfort. Defenses must not be confronted but allowed to operate while they are needed. The nurse can help the client to recognize and talk about fears and misunderstandings. With support and an opportunity to talk, most individuals will gradually come to terms with upsetting information. If the client shows no progress toward accepting the reality of the situation, a referral for additional counseling is advisable.

Sometimes family members insist that the client *not* be told difficult news, such as a diagnosis or test results. They usually have the interests of the client at heart and fear that the news is too painful for the client to bear or will result in depression or giving up. Family members need to know that withholding information will eventually result in the client feeling isolated and sensing that something is wrong.

When the information is received, be prepared for strong *emotions* and remain calm. Let the client know through your words and actions that you are trying to understand his or her feelings. Help the client to express feelings clearly and to use constructive coping strategies. This is a time when empathy is important for the client to believe that you care about the situation.

Anger is a common reaction. It is important to remember that the client is not angry at you but at the situation, and that anger covers up anxiety and disappointment. If you can help the individual express his or her underlying feelings, anger may be diffused. The anger may take the form of blaming you or complaints about care in general. It may be difficult to avoid taking these complaints personally or defending oneself from what seems like a verbal attack. If the individual or significant other feels accepted and comforted, the complaints often decrease or disappear entirely. If the client has a history of violence, alert other staff members that they should be available if needed. Let the client know that you will not allow him or her to hurt him- or herself or others. Set limits on destructive behavior. Let the client know that being destructive with property is not acceptable.

The *summary* is an opportunity to briefly review important information that has been conveyed and to discuss follow-up or what steps need to be taken next. It is important to communicate that there is always hope. Hope may not involve a cure, and the nurse cannot reverse the negative events, but it may be possible to assure the client that everything possible will be done to promote his or her comfort and to support his or her choices at this difficult time.

■ CONCLUSION

Guiding clients through major life experiences such as illness and death is both rewarding and challenging. As you engage in challenging therapeutic interactions, you may wonder if you said the "right" thing. There are no absolute "right" and "wrong" ways to communicate. With supervision and reflection, we can also improve our communication skills. Accepting ourselves and our desire to learn and improve is as important as accepting our clients.

REFERENCES

1. Kotecki, C.N. (2004). Baccalaureate nursing students' communication process in the clinical setting. *Journal of Nursing Education, 41*(2), 61–68.

2. Peplau, H.E. (1952). *Interpersonal relations in nursing.* New York: Putnam.

3. Enslein, J., Tripp-Reimer, T., Kelley, L.S., Choi, E., & McCarty, L. (2002). Evidence-based protocol: Interpreter facilitation for individuals with limited English proficiency. *Journal of Gerontological Nursing, 28*(7), 5–13.

4. Williams, A. (2001). A literature review on the concept of intimacy in nursing. *Journal of Advanced Nursing, 33*(5), 660–667.

5. Williams, C., & Tappen, R. (1999). Can we create a therapeutic relationship with nursing home residents in the later stages of Alzheimer's disease? *Journal of Psychosocial Nursing and Mental Health Services, 37*(3), 1–8.

6. Williams, A., & Irurita, V.F. (2006). Emotional comfort: The patient's perspective of a therapeutic context. *International Journal of Nursing Studies, 43*, 405–415.

7. Radziewicz, R., & Baile, W.F. (2001). Communication skills: Breaking bad news in the clinical setting. *Oncology Nursing Forum, 28*(6), 951–953.

EXERCISES

1. Beginning the Interaction

Opening the conversation requires the use of broad statements or questions that give the client some direction but allows the client freedom to tell his or her "story." Practice writing broad openings as requested below.

Client	Broad Opening from You
I'm here because my sister told me to talk to you about the problems I'm having with my husband. I don't see how it will help.	

2. Asking for Description

Descriptive questions begin with the words "who," "what," "where," and "when." Practice writing descriptive questions as requested below.

Client	Descriptive Questions from You
They told me I had to be admitted to the hospital, but I just want to go home. I felt like hurting myself this morning, but I don't feel that way now.	

3. Open- and Closed-Ended Questions and Statements

Open-ended questions (or statements) cannot be answered with just one word and are more likely to provide rich descriptions from your client. Closed-ended questions can be answered with one word, such as "yes" or "no," and often lead to little or no elaboration by the client. Practice writing open-ended questions and statements by rewording each of the closed-ended questions that follow.

Closed-Ended	Open-Ended
How many children do you have?	Tell me about your family.
Do you think the surgery will help?	
Are you sure you understand the instructions on how to take your medications?	
Do you think you have a drinking problem?	

4. Therapeutic Communication Techniques

Complete the following table with a specific example of the communication technique requested.

Therapeutic Strategy	Client Verbal/Nonverbal Behavior	Your Therapeutic Response
Sharing observations	The client crosses and uncrosses her legs repeatedly during the interview.	"I see that you are restless today. I wonder what is going on?"
General leads	"I think I am dying."	
Identifying themes	The client brings up several arguments with her adolescent son.	
Focusing	Mrs. McArthur, a mother of a 2-year-old, comes to the emergency room because her child has been hurt. After 5 minutes of conversation, you are still not sure how the injury happened.	
Voicing doubt	Based on the physical assessment of her child, Mrs. McArthur's explanation of the child's injuries sounds very unlikely.	
Presenting reality	You present your view of the situation with Mrs. McArthur and her child.	

5

Cross-Cultural Communication

Tamika R. Sanchez-Jones, PhD, MBA, APRN, BC

OBJECTIVES

1. To discuss the importance of communication with diverse populations

2. To examine cultural differences in communication

3. To describe barriers to cross-cultural communication

4. To describe cultural differences in verbal and nonverbal communication

5. To examine individual cultural backgrounds and influence on health care beliefs, values, and behavior

6. To discuss the use of bilingual interpreters to reduce the effects of language barriers

The ability to effectively send and receive messages is essential to communication and allows individuals to interact with each other. This interaction may be especially difficult when the sender and receiver do not share the same cultural background or language. Culture influences how each individual perceives and responds to the world, solves life's problems, and interacts with others. Although there is no single definition of culture, it may be defined as the sum total of behavioral norms, methods of communication, patterns of thinking, and beliefs and values of a designated group of people that can be passed down to the next generation. This may be evident in day-to-day interactions. When shopping or engaging in social activities, you may encounter people who shop in the same stores or wear the same clothes but who look and talk differently than

you. During these interactions, regardless of how brief, there may be awareness of the influence of culture on communication. Differences in communication across cultures are evident in language, verbal and nonverbal behaviors, and silence.[1]

Why is this significant to nursing? When trying to understand the health belief system of a client it is necessary to explore culture. Recent demographic trends indicate increasing cultural and ethnic diversity in the United States leading to a more diverse client population. Within the health care setting, nurses and other providers understand the importance of communication when working with clients. However, there is less understanding of the impact of culture on the communication process. Nurses spend a great deal of their time with clients and therefore must realize the importance of culture as it relates to communication. Transcultural nursing skills and knowledge will be necessary to provide competent care to the rapidly changing, heterogeneous population.

Learning to value cultural and ethnic diversity involves the appreciation of variations in culture as well as negotiating skills for effective communication. Communication with individuals from diverse backgrounds is especially complex because of the influence of culture on language and communication. When communicating with individuals, the nurse should be aware of cultural beliefs and behaviors and communicate (both verbally and nonverbally) in a way that meets the clients' cultural needs. Meeting the needs of clients requires the ability to provide and understand clear and accurate communication.

Intercultural or cross-cultural communication refers to the presence of at least two individuals who are culturally different from each other on important attributes such as value orientations, preferred communication codes, role expectations, and perceived rules of social relationships.[2] Often, speaking the same language does not guarantee understanding between client and nurse.[3] In intercultural communication, differences in communication styles are often met with confusion, impatience, and misunderstanding. Imagine how difficult it would be to communicate when the listener does not share the same language, context, or symbolism. How could you teach a newly diagnosed insulin-dependent diabetic about dietary management and medication regimens when there is not a shared language or culture? How could you assist in developing menu plans when you are unaware of culturally specific foods? How could you explain the use of insulin and the procedure for administration if you do not speak the language? These issues represent the difficulties in intercultural communication. Table 5-1 offers guidelines for cross-cultural communication.

Although knowledge of cultural rules and norms can help to avoid mistakes in communication, it is not possible for individuals to be familiar or competent with the differences in communication patterns for all cultures. Even when you are aware of cultural differences, it is difficult to consider the subtle differences among individuals within the same culture. Nurses must be open to subgroup variability within cultures. Differences may be seen within the culture based on factors such as gender,

educational level, income, and status. Additionally, recognize and apologize for mistakes in communication to maintain trust and respect for communication.[4]

■ OVERCOMING BARRIERS TO PROVIDING CROSS-CULTURAL CARE

When caring for clients from diverse populations, nurses should be aware of their own cultural behaviors and habits. Each individual is socialized into a cultural environment. Assuming cultures are similar to your own will lead to confusion and misinterpretation of messages. It is better to expect differences and explore ways in which these differences will affect communication. Nurses may have little awareness of how their own cultural beliefs define the type of care they give or messages they send to clients. Both nonverbal and verbal communication skills are important in the nursing process. How would a client from a different culture respond to personal questions regarding health practices or personal history? How do others perceive personal uses of distance, gestures, and dialect? Cultural differences in both verbal and nonverbal communication will be discussed later in this chapter.

Cultural barriers may also be present in the way in which members of an ethnic group perceive health, illness, and discharge following treatment.[5] Effective communication is the ability to understand the other person's perspective. For example, clients who view illness as a punishment or curse may delay medical treatment or seek medical treatment only as a last resort.

Table 5-1   Guidelines for Cross-Cultural Communication

Do	Do not
1. Be aware of your own cultural beliefs and biases	1. Stereotype
2. Be open to learning more about the other person's communication style	2. Assume there is only one way to communicate (yours)
3. Practice engaging in cross-cultural communication	3. Assume that breakdowns in communication are due to the other person's errors
4. Listen actively and allow time for cross-cultural communication	4. Presume communication means understanding
5. Respect the other person's decision to engage in communication with you	5. Assume all cultures are similar to yours
6. Explore speech patterns of the group	
7. Be aware of nonverbal communication	
8. Clarify messages	
9. Be aware that communication occurs in context	

Source: Adapted from Smith-Trudeau, P. (2001). Communication guarantees nothing. *Vermont Nurses Connection, 4*(4), 1, 3.

Respect for cultural traditions will take into account alternative health care practices and beliefs such as the use of lay practitioners and complementary therapies while incorporating medical interventions.

Ethnocentric values may make it difficult for the nurse to be objective in providing care, especially to diverse populations. Ethnocentrism is the belief that one's own culture is superior to that of another.[6] Being proud of one's own culture is appropriate, but the difficulty begins when there is less respect for the values or beliefs of the other person. Listen to the client's view with an open mind. The nurse should refrain from defending or imparting their own cultural beliefs.[4] For example, instead of trying to understand a newly admitted client from the client's cultural context, the ethnocentric nurse would try to understand the client within the nurse's own cultural context. Nurses should respect the differences in behavior and knowledge that may influence health care practices and recognize that their own ideas or behavior may not be best for every client.[7] Ethnocentrism may make it difficult for the nurse to accept client decisions not based on the nurse's culturally derived value system or beliefs.

Case example

Mr. Rodriquez, a 65-year-old Hispanic male, was admitted at 8:00 p.m. to the hospital following a stroke. Visiting hours were just ending, and Mr. Rodriquez was accompanied by his wife and four grown children and their spouses. The nurse felt overwhelmed with so many relatives present, but they were insistent that they needed to stay with the client through the night. What would be the nurse's most appropriate course of action?

■ HIGH- AND LOW-CONTEXT CULTURES

Hall[8] conceptualized high- and low-context cultures. When individuals attempt to communicate, it is important to understand the amount of information transmitted through words versus the context of the situation. Context refers to the situation and/or environment where the communication occurs and helps to define the communication. Culture is also considered to be context and may set the stage for communication. However, cultures may differ in the amount and type of information conveyed through verbal and nonverbal cues.

In intercultural interactions, there are differences in high- and low-context communication patterns. Individuals from high-context cultures rely on an understanding of shared experiences without the need for many words. There is meaning attached to the context, and there is more communication contained in the context of the situation vs the words spoken. Emphasis is placed on nonverbal interactions such as nonverbal cues and messages.[9,10] People from high-context cultures consider themselves part of the larger group and value shared experiences. There is also an appreciation for history and tradition.

One example of high-context culture is your own family environment. When communicating with individuals with whom you are familiar, such as family members, there is little need for explanations or highly detailed information. In high-context cultures, there is a familiarity with one another and minimal verbal communication is needed to gain understanding. In those situations, even facial expressions can communicate complex messages. There is an underlying message or metaphoric association in the communication.[11] For example, you probably knew your mother was displeased by your behavior with just a look or you can signal approval for a friend's new outfit with a wink or the thumbs up gesture. There is little need for your mother to give you a detailed explanation of her disapproval of your behavior, and a friend would clearly understand your nonverbal communication without the need for clarification. Asians, Saudi Arabians, Spanish, Africans, African Americans, Mexican Americans, and Native Americans engage in high-context communication.

In the case example, the nurse, recognizing that Mr. Rodriquez is part of a high-context cultural group, will understand the value he places on being part of a group and sharing important experiences with the group. Nonverbal communication is facilitated when family members are present. In this situation the nurse would be creative and flexible about including family members while respecting the needs of other clients.

Cultures engaged in low-context communication use more words and are impatient with others who do not make themselves understood quickly. Meaning is derived from the message. There is little meaning attached to the context. Verbal messages are elaborate, highly detailed, and redundant. Low-context cultures lack shared meanings and continuity. The ability to make oneself understood is valued. Individuals from low-context cultures may not understand the use of gestures and nonverbal cues that are frequently used in high-context cultures.[9] Low-context communication is best described by the type of communication one would have with a stranger where you would have to explain ideas in detail because there may be no shared understanding or experiences. Silence and other nonverbal cues may be confusing and irritating to low-context communicators. Those from low-context cultures include Anglo-Europeans, Canadians, European Americans, and Germans.

When communication is attempted between individuals from high-context and low-context cultures, the high-context communicator offers little information or clarity and utilizes silence and nonverbal cues to encourage understanding. This may be very frustrating to those from a low-context culture. In contrast, the low-context communicator offers elaborate explanations, which may lead the high-context communicator to believe that they are not being understood.

■ VERBAL COMMUNICATION

Not only do we base our opinions of others on verbal communication, but we also attempt to define social status and emotions on the way individuals speak and make themselves understood. Communication patterns, pitch, and rate differ among cultures. African Americans share and express feelings openly to family members and close friends. The pitch may be fast and the tone loud and confrontational. For European Americans, the pitch is slower and the tone is nonchallenging and less personal. Asians are typically soft-spoken and do not challenge during conversation. Muslim or Arabic speech tends to be repetitive and exaggerated. Displays of emotion represent a deep concern for the topic of discussion.

The discussion of personal issues with strangers is considered inappropriate within the African American, Arabian, and Asian cultures. In contrast, Latinos will usually appreciate inquiries about family members. In the health care setting, variations in verbal communication may be evident while trying to take a health history or attempting to understand the religious practices of an African American client. African Americans believe in prayer to promote health and well-being. African Americans may also "speak in tongues," a prayer that is understood only by the person speaking, and therefore this display of prayer and spirituality may be confusing for individuals from other cultures. Asians, Middle Easterners and Latin Americans seek to "save face" at all costs.

The dignity of these clients must be preserved at all times to avoid "loss of face." Nurses need to be particularly sensitive to avoid humiliation or inadvertent slights to clients from these cultures.[12]

Regional, racial, and ethnic accents are also important and may lead to assumptions or stereotyping. The accents and speech patterns of urban minority youths may be perceived negatively by educated Anglo-Europeans. What other types of accents or regional dialects can you identify that are associated with strong assumptions?

■ NONVERBAL COMMUNICATION

It is often said that "actions speak louder than words," and this may be especially true when communicating across cultures. Nonverbal communication can be defined as the deliberate or unintentional use of touch, distance, space, gestures, and time to communicate meaning. These messages may indicate approval, status, emotion, and power. Effective communication considers not only the spoken word but also the nonverbal nuances. Additional forms of nonverbal communication not discussed in this section include e-mail, clothing, tattoos, and artifacts (physical objects such as cars, jewelry, etc.).

Touch

Touch is a meaningful form of nonverbal communication.[13] The amount and type of touch may differ related to gender, age, socioeconomic factors, and individual preferences.[9] Touch can indicate emotions from approval and comfort to aggression and anger. For example, patting someone on the back can indicate approval or acceptance in many cultures while touching someone with the left hand is considered inappropriate and disrespectful among Muslims. In addition, for strict Muslims and Orthodox Jews, a handshake between men and women in a public setting is inappropriate and considered to be disrespectful.

Mexican and Native Americans believe that touch is magical and healing. Within the Vietnamese culture, touch may provoke anxiety because it is thought to release the soul from the body.[7] Touching the head, even of a small child, may be viewed as offensive to some Asians. African Americans and Hispanics tend to be comfortable with close personal space and frequent touch while interacting with close friends and relatives.

Handshaking is a generally accepted greeting in America, especially in business. The type and length of a handshake differs across cultures. In America the handshake is firm. In Asia the handshake is soft with the other hand brought up underneath to signify warmth and friendship. In contrast, many Latin Americans see the handshake as impersonal and distant. Hispanics may greet friends, family, and acquaintances with an embrace.

Culture influences the amount and type of physical contact that is considered to be acceptable. It is usually a good idea to ask questions and explain the reason for touch, such as physical examination, prior to initiating the touch. Be open to feedback and adapt your behavior as necessary.

Distance

The amount of distance and space highly influences the message sent to others. The amount of space differs among cultures and may also vary within cultures based on gender and other variables. Familiarity and trust may also determine the comfortable distance. Regardless of cultural background we each have some sense of discomfort when others are "in our space." Are there people who make you uncomfortable because they invade your space? Do you notice that people often step backward or step toward you when you are attempting to communicate?

The nature of relationships is conveyed through the use of personal zones. Hall[14] defines extensions of personal space across cultures, and the following zones define these distances:

- Intimate zone—Touching to 18 inches occurs during private situations. This distance is best for assessing breath and body odors. When this space is invaded by others than those that are emotionally close, we feel threatened. Visual distortions also occur in this zone, and the voice may be at a whisper.

- Personal zone—Eighteen inches to 4 feet occurs most often as the distance during a handshake. Also, this is the distance most couples stand in public. The voice is moderate, body odor is not apparent, and there are no physical distortions. The physical examination typically occurs at this distance.

- Social/causal zone—Four feet to 8 feet occurs during impersonal business transactions. Interviews occur at this distance.

- Public zone—Beyond 8 feet occurs in situations such as teaching and other less personal interactions.

The speaker must project his or her voice, and it is difficult to assess facial expression due to distance.

Hispanics and Asians typically prefer less distance and stand closer to each other than do Anglo-Europeans. The nurse should also be aware that many cultures prefer that same sex healthcare providers perform intimate physical and mental examinations. The nurse should try to meet the client's request to preserve client modesty and participation.

When working with clients who prefer more personal space, the nurse may sit in a chair at the end of the bed in an acute care setting or in a chair opposite the client in a community or clinic setting. When less distance is desired, the nurse may sit at the head of the bed or closer to the client.

Gestures

Gestures can also communicate messages and cues to others. Expressions of self through body movements can facilitate and enhance communication. Head nodding, pointing, smiles, and general body movements can help to clarify other forms of communication, and they vary among cultures. In a number of cultures, nodding of the head signifies agreement. However, within the Japanese culture head nodding is indicative of attentiveness, not agreement, and could be easily misunderstood.[14] Pointing as in summoning a waiter is commonplace in American society while in other cultures it is considered to be rude.

Emotions may also be influenced by culture. While Americans may openly laugh or smile when happy or amused, Asians may laugh or smile when speaking of unpleasant or embarrassing situations. Koreans, in contrast, believe that laughing and frequent smiling demonstrates unintelligence and therefore they are often serious under most circumstances.

Eye Contact

Patterns of eye contact differ across cultures. Eye contact communicates respect, status, and regulates turn-taking in a conversation in American society. In American society one may look away or avoid direct eye contact when they are embarrassed or uncomfortable in a situation. Think back to a time when you may have avoided direct eye contact when a professor posed a question to which you did not know the answer.

A direct stare by African Americans or Arabians is not intended as a threat or a sign of rudeness, while an indirect gaze or downward gaze is seen as a sign of respect among most Asians.

Time

Attempting to communicate across cultural barriers requires knowledge by the nurse of the differences in the perception of time. Have you ever noticed how some people are always late regardless of the situation while others are punctual to a fault? The perception of time varies among cultures. Time orientation determines if members of a cultural group view time in the present, past, or future. Cultures that are future oriented plan long term and are readily accepting of health care regimens to prevent future illness. They keep appointments more often and engage in health promotion activities. Clients who are oriented to the present show less concern for health care regimens and are less likely to keep or be on time for appointments.[1]

A shared belief by African Americans and Mexican Americans is that time is flexible and that events do not begin until they arrive. This may be problematic when scheduling appointments and follow-ups. The nurse who is aware of this cultural variation will allow some flexibility when planning care for these clients.

■ UTILIZING BILINGUAL TRANSLATORS

There may be situations when you must confront differences in both culture and language. This may become very difficult when explaining a diagnosis or trying to obtain informed consent for a medical treatment. Although most health care institutions offer some type of service and/or provide staff to meet the needs of culturally diverse patients, nurses can be effective in preparing themselves for the interaction. Using interpreters can assist nurses in communication across language barriers. When there are no formally trained interpreters available, a bilingual family member may serve as an available interpreter only at the request and approval of the client. Federal HIPAA guidelines offer privacy and confidentiality protection to all clients even if they are not able to understand their rights.

Often children are used to interpret because they are usually more proficient in the second language. Par-

ents, children, or close friends and family members may censor or be reluctant to share personal or intimate matters because of embarrassment. While it may be convenient to use family members, clients may also be less willing to disclose personal information and therefore make the nurse–client relationship difficult and awkward. Family members may also have limited knowledge of the content needed to adequately relate health information and instructions. Complex medical terminology and explanations may be difficult. Additionally, family members may be reluctant to share sensitive or bad news with the client.

Due to the sensitive issues often discussed in the nurse–patient relationship, the use of children as interpreters is discouraged. When possible the use of professionally trained, same sex interpreters is preferred. In addition, it is recommended that the nurse meet with the interpreter to review the goals and purposes of the meeting with the family. It is also a good idea for the interpreter to meet with the family to prepare for the session as well as establish rapport. The nurse should speak directly to the client and family during the session and not to the interpreter. Avoiding complicating medical jargon and keeping answers simple and concrete help to avoid mishaps in translation. Also allow plenty of time for the interpreter to relay information and encourage questions when appropriate. The use of good interpreters is an invaluable resource to nurses and the health care team.[15]

■ CONCLUSION

The ability to communicate both verbally and nonverbally to diverse populations is crucial to providing effective transcultural care. A culturally sensitive nurse seeks to incorporate knowledge of the client's culture in providing therapeutic nursing care. Lack of effective communication may impede the nursing process when working with diverse clients. Cultural and language differences do not need to pose barriers to providing nursing care. The greater your understanding of communication patterns of diverse cultures, the more effective your ability to communicate. Practice and more practice are essential to increase competence in cross-cultural communication.

REFERENCES

1. Spector, R.E. (2003). *Cultural diversity in health and illness/culture care: Guide to heritage assessment health* (5th ed.). Upper Saddle River, NJ: Prentice Hall Health.

2. Lustig, M.W., & Koester, J. (2005). *Intercultural competence: Interpersonal communication across cultures.* New York: Addison Wesley.

3. Tate, D.M. (2003). Cultural awareness: Bridging the gap between caregivers and Hispanic patients. *Journal of Continuing Education in Nursing, 34*(5), 213–217.

4. Anonymous. (2004). Bridging gaps in cross-cultural communication. *Tar Heel Nurse, 66*(2), 15.

5. Betchel, G.A., & Davidhizar, R. (2002). A cultural assessment model for ED patients. *Journal of Emergency Nursing, 25*(5), 377–380.

6. Leininger, M., & MacFarland, M.R. (2005). *Cultural care diversity and universality: A worldwide nursing theory.* Boston: Jones & Bartlett.

7. Giger, J.N., & Davidhizar, R.E. (2004). *Transcultural nursing: Assessment and intervention.* St. Louis, MO: Mosby.

8. Hall, E.T. (1976). *Beyond culture.* New York: Doubleday.

9. Lynch, E.W., & Hanson, M.J. (2004). *Developing cross-cultural competence: A guide for working with children and their families* (3rd ed.). Baltimore: Paul H. Brookes.

10. Harris, P., Moran, R., & Moran, S. (2004). *Managing cultural differences.* Philadelphia: Butterworth-Heinemann.

11. Kabagarama, D. (1999). *Breaking the ice: A guide to understanding people from other cultures.* New York: Prentice Hall.

12. Gardenswartz, L., & Rowe, A. (1998). *Managing diversity in health care.* San Francisco: Jossey-Bass.

13. DeFleur, M.H., Kearney, P., Plax, T.G., & DeFleur, M.L. (2004). *Fundamentals of human communication.* Boston: McGraw-Hill.

14. Hall, E.T. (1959). *The silent language.* New York: Doubleday.

15. Lum, D. (2003). *Social work practice and people of color: A process-stage approach.* Belmont, CA: Wadsworth Thomas.

EXERCISES

A. Review and answer each question independently, and then compare your answers with someone within your family, and then discuss with a group of friends or colleagues.

> When you were a child, what were the health care beliefs and behaviors of your family?
>
> What did your family do to stay healthy?
>
> What did your family believe caused illness?
>
> How were specific illnesses treated?
>
> Who was responsible for deciding the appropriate treatment?
>
> What health care practitioners outside of the family were used to treat illness?

1. How are the answers to the questions similar and/or different from your family members?

2. How are the answers to the questions similar and/or different from your friends or colleagues?

3. What surprised you the most while completing this exercise?

B. Examine your personal beliefs about the following cultural groups. How might your personal beliefs and values affect your ability to communicate with individuals from each of the cultural groups? You may choose to do this privately so that you may be honest with your answers.

Mexican Americans

Africans

Chinese Americans

Japanese Americans

European Americans

Cuban Americans

African Americans

Navajos

6

Communicating with Families

Christine L. Williams, DNSc, APRN, BC and Tamika R. Sanchez-Jones, PhD, MBA, APRN, BC

OBJECTIVES

1. To compare communication with individual clients to family-focused communication

2. To discuss how cultural traditions may influence interactions with families

3. To describe strategies for communicating with families

■ INTRODUCTION

Nurses have traditionally conceptualized their care as family centered. In the past most nursing care was delivered in hospital settings where family members' access to nurses was limited by visiting hours and rigid rules for interaction. In this era of community-based care, effective communication with families is becoming increasingly important. More care is delivered in ambulatory and home settings where nurses have frequent contact with families.

■ FAMILY COMPOSITION

For purposes of developing relationships that support clients' recovery, the term "family" is loosely defined. Nontraditional families may include members who are not blood or legal relatives yet they live with and have strong emotional ties to the client. Clients may identify a same sex partner as their closest relative. Not everyone has living relatives who are available to help them during illness.

> Mrs. James, age 89, is the last living member of a large family. Her closest "family member" is Hazel, her neighbor and long-time friend of 30 years. When Mrs. James is hospitalized, Hazel is designated as her health care proxy.

Family members may not live with the client but may be very involved in their care. Sometimes caregivers live in a distant state (or even another country) but would like more communication with nurses about their loved one's care. Caregivers may work full time during regular business hours and would welcome communication with nurses about their loved one's care.

Many patients and families experience difficulty in communicating with nurses and other health professionals.[1] Communication between nurses and family members is often infrequent and fragmented.

> Mrs. Jackson works full time as a high school teacher and has little time during working hours to use the telephone. Her mother is a resident in a nearby nursing facility. Mrs. Jackson visits twice a week, once on Wednesday evenings and again on Saturdays. She has no communication with nurses or other health professionals at the facility. She receives written invitations to periodic interdisciplinary meetings regarding her mother's care, but the meetings are always scheduled during her work hours. She sees the same nurses when she visits her mother but they always seem so busy and never initiate conversation about how her mother is doing.

■ WHOSE RESPONSIBILITY IS IT TO COMMUNICATE WITH FAMILY MEMBERS?

Nurses have frequently viewed communication with the family as the physician's or the social worker's responsibility. Too often, family members are not included in the client's care, and communication with the family is neglected. Regardless of who the client identifies as family, it is important to maintain communication. Family members can provide vital information about the client. Children, cognitively impaired individuals, and very sick clients may not be able to provide a history, and the family member may be the only source of information. Building an alliance with family members can make the difference between success and failure of the care plan. They can either support or undermine your efforts to positively impact the client's health.

■ HOW IS FAMILY-CENTERED COMMUNICATION DIFFERENT FROM COMMUNICATION WITH INDIVIDUALS?

Communicating with families generally implies communicating with more than one person. Interaction with a group requires different skills than communicating with individuals one at a time. Families have customary ways of communicating. There are alliances and rules for interaction between members that will influence decision making and the flow of information. How do families normally exchange information among members? To answer this question, begin by noticing family members' nonverbal communication. Who contacts you to set up a meeting or to ask for information? In a meeting with the family, who sits next to whom? Who speaks to whom? Who seems to speak for the group?

Confidentiality can become a challenge when several family members want to be involved in the client's care. You will need to carefully consider who should receive confidential information. If clients are able to decide who should receive information, the nurse can rely on their instructions. When clients have diminished capacity to make decisions, the nurse will rely on state laws regarding who has the legal right to act as a proxy. Although you may not disclose information without appropriate permission, you can still meet with the family to allow them to express their concerns and emotions and provide you with information about the client. Some families may not want the client to receive details of a diagnosis or facts about the severity of their illness.

They may be concerned that the truth will result in despair and the client will give up prematurely. Such dilemmas should be discussed with the interdisciplinary team or may have to be resolved by an ethics committee.

When interacting with a family, there is increased risk of misunderstandings and miscommunication. To minimize these problems, try to gather the family in one place and give information once. If you must interact with only one person, be aware that the designated person may not disseminate information to other family members accurately and completely. It is best not to assume that one member will take care of all family communication.

> Mrs. Rodriquez (age 85) was hospitalized for repair of a fractured hip. Mrs. Rodriquez's daughter, Maria (age 55), visited her mother daily. When the nurse tried to initiate discussion of discharge plans for her mother, Maria was vague and noncommittal. On the weekend, Mrs. Rodriguez's son visited and began asking about discharge plans. It became clear that Maria was not the decision maker and was waiting for her brother to visit.

Respect boundaries between family subgroups. In families of older adults, support the integrity of the spousal relationship. Children (regardless of age) should not be given important information before a spouse. The spouse is the appropriate person with whom to communicate. Special circumstances such as a spouse's illness or lack of cognitive capacity will necessarily alter your plan for communicating. When a spouse is severely impaired, the health care proxy becomes the person with whom you will communicate. In families with younger children, parents are obviously your point of contact. Even this family structure may present communication challenges. Divorce, custody disputes, and joint custody arrangements may create barriers to communication with family members. Adolescents should be included with the parents in discussions of their care.

The Family Meeting

Successful communication during a family meeting begins with preparation. Whenever possible, ask the client or resident who should be included. Sometimes clients are too young or too ill to provide direction. In the case of older adults and their adult children, they often come into the health care setting together. Find out if this is the client's next of kin and who else can or should be included. The need to balance inclusion of family members in communication and protection of the client's privacy can create dilemmas for the nurse. Questions about who to include can be discussed with the health care team.

Consideration of the communication environment can convey respect for the family. In a health care facility, it is your responsibility to provide adequate seating with as much privacy as possible. Sit at the same level as the family members to communicate equality. Avoid sitting behind a barrier such as a desk. When client and family members are present in a meeting together, the nurse needs to address the client directly rather than speak about the client as if she or he were not in the room. To convey the message "I value you," ask for opinions and input from everyone present. If family members seem to want you to take sides in disputes, remain neutral to not alienate one side or the other. Recognize their efforts to be there and to be involved in the care.

Be cautious if a family member asks to confide a secret and asks that you refrain from sharing information with the client or other members of the health team. Never promise to keep information from the health team, especially when you have not heard the content of the secret.

The Role of Setting

The decision about who to communicate with varies according to the situation and setting. Generally long-term settings and life threatening situations require more family interaction. When we establish long-term relationships with clients (such as admission to long-term care, home care, or hospice care), the involvement of supportive others is critical to obtaining a complete assessment and laying the foundation for cooperation and trust. When the setting is a health care environment (such as a rehabilitation unit), subtle nonverbal communication can make the difference in whether or not the nurse establishes a successful relationship. Who does the nurse make eye contact with when speaking? Who is encouraged to be present as care is administered and who is asked to leave the room? Does the nurse extend visiting times for some family members and not for others? How many family members are too many? Who should be included when there is bad news? All of these questions should be considered and discussed with colleagues involved in the care of the client and family. Consistency in communication and in approach to the family will help to ensure cooperation and minimize dissatisfaction with care.

When the setting for a family meeting is the home, advance planning is important. Choose a time when as many family members as possible are available. Notice what the living arrangements tell you about how the family functions. If you are invited to tour the home, take this opportunity to see how the family uses their living space. Do the living arrangements convey concern for the quality of life of the client and other members of the family? If you are offered something to eat or drink, refusing may be interpreted as a rejection of their hospitality. In the home setting, the nurse is the guest and the family has more control over who attends the meeting and who participates. Notice who seems most involved and interested and who can be counted on for participation in the client's care.

■ COMMUNICATING WITH LATINO/HISPANIC FAMILIES

Latinos/Hispanics now represent 14.5% of the U.S. population and are the fastest growing minority group. The Hispanic population is diverse. Hispanics represent many countries and races with different backgrounds and traditions.[2] Although stereotyping can be problematic and every family will differ in how much they conform to cultural traditions, some generalizations are helpful to formulate an initial approach to a particular Hispanic family. Cultural traditions can have an important impact on communication with families. As with any group, labels are important. Latino and Hispanic are terms used to describe those who trace their family ancestry to a Spanish speaking country. Hispanic is a term that may be offensive to some because it is associated with a history of colonization by the Spanish. Latino is associated with Latin American heritage. Individuals who are not from Latin America may prefer to be designated Hispanic rather than Latino (such as Cuban Americans).[3] For purposes of this discussion the label "Hispanic" will be used to mean Latino, Latina, or Hispanic.

Some traditions and values such as *familismo* are important to most Hispanics. Family cohesiveness, or familismo, is a value that plays a critical role in how Hispanic families communicate. Familismo means that Hispanics value the welfare of the family over the needs of the individual. Their focus on interdependence and a traditional patriarchal hierarchy usually results in frequent contact among family members and sharing of information. The nurse should communicate with the family as a group or with the highest ranking family member.[3] Although the highest ranking family member in the traditional Hispanic family is often the eldest male,[4] the number of female heads of household is increasing rapidly.[3] Out of respect for authority and family hierarchy, the client may want to consult with the family decision maker before health care decisions are made. Hispanic families have a strong tradition of caring for their family members in times of illness even at the expense of their own health. Advising a family member to get outside help with caregiving may not be welcomed and will likely be ignored.[4]

Health care professionals value transparency in communication. They have been taught that sharing as much information as is available is usually best for the client. This belief may conflict with the family's unspoken rules about withholding information if they believe it is in the client's best interest. For example, if the nurse communicates openly with a client about issues such as death and dying, he or she may come in conflict with the head of the family, who would prefer that such information be withheld from the client.

Compared to mainstream American families, extended family is likely to be more involved in the client's care. Extended family members play an important role in providing both emotional support and help with instrumental tasks.[4] Although it may not be feasible to maintain ongoing communication with all extended family members, the nurse needs to facilitate their presence, encourage their help, and recognize the key role of specific members such as grandparents.

Hispanics value warm, personal relationships (*personalismo*) more than formal relationships that adhere to rules and regulations. This means that the family will expect you to spend some time in friendly conversation before beginning to discuss the purpose of your visit. Insisting on adhering to a strict agenda for a conversation may be interpreted as rude. Your warmth and friendliness will engender rapport. If you want your clients to trust you, be attentive to this tradition. Patients may tend to be more formal initially, so a formal greeting is more appropriate at first. With the client's permission, a more familiar address may be used later. Older adults are always shown more respect, so use a formal address for older adults in the family.[3]

Another cultural tradition "*simpatica*"[3] is the desire to be pleasing in relationships. An informal tone is generally most comfortable in a meeting. "Cuban people are gregarious and come from a cheerful culture attributable to the Caribbean influence. A visit may be more relaxed than most while still accomplishing care goals."[4]

Hispanics may have limited proficiency in English. Many prefer to speak Spanish at home.[3] A nurse from the same background is desirable. Even when speaking Spanish, the speaker needs to be aware of nonverbal cues such as the pace of speech. "Spanish is spoken quickly, but requests should be made slowly so as not to be perceived as forceful."[4]

■ COMMUNICATING WITH AFRICAN AMERICAN FAMILIES

African Americans represent the second largest minority group in the United States, second to Hispanics, and account for 12.3% of the U.S. population.[2] In the United States, African American or the term "black" is used to describe individuals who trace their ancestors to Africa, recent immigrants from Africa, Jamaicans, Haitians, etc. For the purposes of this discussion, African American will be used to describe individuals who trace their ancestry back through slavery to Africa.

The African American culture is diverse while many African Americans are deeply rooted in African American life and traditions. African Americans value family and have strong, extended support systems that provide support and assistance during illness. African Americans value respect for elders and female family members. African Americans tend to be more inclusive when selecting individuals to be involved in health care decisions. Extended family and nonkin "relatives" are also included in decision making. Health care decisions and problems are often solved using a group approach.[5]

While many families in the United States are headed by males (patriarchal), the impact of slavery on the male as protector and provider in the African American family continues to be problematic. African American families are often matriarchal, and the female is often considered to be the highest ranking family member and must be consulted prior to making health care decisions. African American women tend to provide direct care for family members in times of illness and are often trapped in the "sandwich generation" caring for aging parents and ill family members while raising their own children and working full time. The nurse must be aware of the importance of the African American female in decision making while still respecting the presence of other family members when disseminating information and assisting with decision making. While nurses should encourage family members to seek assistance in providing care, seeking outside assistance or government intervention is often seen as a weakness and a violation of privacy.

African Americans perceive illness as a natural occurrence and accept illness as God's will. Often, illness may be seen as a result of an uncontrollable event (cold weather, voodoo, environmental hazards) or punishment (sins, unemployment, spiritual problems). Folk medicine and nontraditional health practices are a common occurrence, especially in the South, and have been passed down from African tradition and practices during slavery. Nontraditional health practices include the use of parsley tea for urinary tract infections or castor oil to treat minor illnesses.

African Americans may speak what is often referred to as "black English," which is often spoken quickly and uses words distorted from standard English. Speech is typically very graphic and rhythmic, accompanied by expressive body movements and facial expressions. Although grammatically different from standard English, black English should not be viewed as inferior or substandard.[6] Nurses should be aware that many African Americans are adept at duality of speech and can switch from black English to standard English depending on who they are communicating with.

▪ SUMMARY

Family caregivers play a vital role in maintaining the health of chronically ill elders, disabled clients, and chronically ill children. Families of ill clients need the opportunity to share their experiences, talk about their anxieties and their losses, and learn to communicate about difficult emotions with their ill family members.[7] A nurse who is comfortable talking to families can facilitate their help, minimize misunderstandings, and promote the client's comfort and recovery through stressful experiences.

REFERENCES

1. Dunne, K. (2005). Effective communication in palliative care. *Nursing Standard, 20*(13), 57–64.

2. U.S. Bureau of the Census (2005). *2005 American community survey data profile highlights.* Retrieved March 30, 2007, from http://factfinder.census.gov/servlet/ACSSAFFFacts?_submenuId=factsheet_0&_sse=on.

3. Smith, T.B. (2004). *Practicing multiculturalism: Affirming diversity in counseling and psychology.* Boston: Pearson.

4. Smith, R.L., & Montilla, R.E. (2006). *Counseling and family therapy with Latino populations: Strategies that work.* New York: Routledge.

5. Rodriguez, J. (1998). Culture tips: Cuban-Americans. *Cross Cultural Connection, 4*(1), 5.

6. Waites, C., Macgowan, M., Pennell, J., Carlton-LaNey, C., & Weil, M. (2004). Increasing the cultural responsiveness of family group conferencing. *Social Work, 49*(2), 291–300.

7. Giger, J., & Davidhiar, R. (2004). *Transcultural nursing: Assessment and intervention.* St. Louis, MO: Mosby.

8. Walton-Moss, B., Gerson, L., & Ross, L. (2005). Effects of mental illness on family quality of life. *Issues in Mental Health Nursing, 26,* 627–642.

Exercises

1. Self-Assessment

Some clients (children, older clients) are likely to be accompanied by family members in health care situations. Communicating with families is more complicated than dealing with individuals alone. Use the following exercises to explore your communication with families.

A. Think about how you learned to communicate in your family of origin (the family you grew up in). How would you describe your family's patterns of communication?

When I had good news, I usually shared it with

When I had a problem, I liked to talk to

When things went wrong in our family, we handled it by

How did your family's cultural background affect verbal and nonverbal communication among members?

B. Think about how you communicate in your family now. How would you describe your family's patterns of communication?

I usually share good news with

When I have a problem, I like to talk to

When things went wrong in our family, we communicated by

How comfortable are you talking with family members?

How does culture affect the way your family responds to challenges?

How do you usually communicate with families in the clinical setting?

What was the most challenging experience you have had communicating with a family?

Discussion

Do you prefer to work with clients one to one or with clients and families? What factors influence your preferences? In your self-assessment notebook, summarize what you have learned in doing these exercises.

2. Responding to Situations

A. You are a nurse in a nursing home. One of the residents on your unit has a daughter who visits daily after work. A son who lives in another state telephones often. They usually seek you out to complain about their father's care. You believe that their complaints are unfounded.

What might your feelings be in this situation?

What would you really like to say to the resident's daughter?

What could you say that might be therapeutic?

B. You are a nurse in the neonatal intensive care unit. You are assigned to care for a neonate who is critically ill. The parents are present most of the time. The baby's parents are talking together quietly. You approach them to offer support.

What can you say or do to communicate your support during this difficult time?

Section 3
Communicating
in Special Circumstances

7

Communicating with Children

Lois S. Marshall, PhD, RN, CPN

OBJECTIVES

1. To describe the development of language as a means of communication

2. To discuss normal communication patterns of children of various ages

3. To discuss strategies that the nurse can use to enhance communication with children

Once upon a time, a small rabbit was lost in a maze. The rabbit searched and circled looking for a way to his destination. During the trip, the rabbit came across a giraffe. The rabbit came up to the giraffe's big toenail. The giraffe asked the rabbit if help was needed. The rabbit looked up tentatively and somewhat awed with the size of the giraffe. The rabbit took two steps backward and looked up . . . way up . . . way, way up. With trepidation, the rabbit said, "No thank you," and started to move away.

Such is the communication between children and nurses who tower over them. Nurses look different than children, just as the giraffe looks different from the rabbit. The differences in appearance, size, and development will affect the communication patterns between nurses and children. These differences must be addressed to better understand normal communication patterns of children of different ages and cognitive levels. For nurses to communicate with children effectively, the rabbit and giraffe scenario must be avoided by adapting communication techniques to the appropriate level of the children they are caring for.

■ FAMILY-CENTERED COMMUNICATION

Communication with children is family centered. It is a process involving the nurse, parent(s) or caregiver, and child.[1] In today's society of expanded and nontraditional families, there may be many other participants in the communication process, and nurses should note that the principles of communication with families are the same regardless of family makeup.

Although nurses must communicate with both child and family members to be effective as health care providers, the age and cognitive development of the child dictate how much communication will take place with all members of the family present and when separate discussions might be more appropriate. Nurses working with children must have knowledge of family dynamics, relationships, cultural differences, and established communication patterns within the family structure. It is knowledge of how the family communicates that will best assist the nurse in determining the ideal strategy for communicating with the child separately and as an active, participating member of the family.

■ COMMUNICATION IN CHILDREN

For children, communication is a process that evolves as cognition, physical and psychosocial development, and experience increase. Communication takes practice and repetition, interaction with role models, confidence, as well as verbal and nonverbal skills. As early as gestation, humans participate in varying forms of communication. Prospective parents listen to classical music, talk to their baby, and read books to "mommy's tummy" in hopes that these forms of language are heard, even at a very basic level.

From infancy through adolescence, communication is a dynamic, ongoing, ever-changing, and constantly developing process. Communication continues as the infant begins to interact with the environment and the people in it. Somatic language[2] is primarily the language of infants' communication, although components of this means of communication can continue throughout one's lifespan. Somatic language is focused on communicating through nonverbal vocalization, such as crying to make an infant's needs heard; facial expressions, as when an infant grimaces and spits out a new food that tastes bad; jerking movements; and the reddening of skin, as in frustration in an infant, which in later life is often identified as blushing with embarrassment. Action language[2] begins later in infancy as the child learns to communicate wants and needs by reaching, pointing, crawling toward or away, turning his or her head, and/or closing his or her lips. The infant's ability to communicate is guided by what these actions mean to him- or herself and how these actions are interpreted by the caregiver. Verbal language,[2] while beginning with the first spoken word at 6 to 7 months of age, does not really become an effective means of communication until toddlerhood. The toddler's language development progresses from repetitive noises and sounds to word usage, to phrase usage, and finally to sentence usage. This process grows and becomes more refined with experience and cognitive development throughout one's lifetime.

■ COMMUNICATION AND COGNITIVE DEVELOPMENT

The younger infant, age 1 to 6 months, uses primarily nonverbal communication. The infant responds to adults through tactile stimulation and by the sound and tone of the adult's voice. At this age, the infant uses vocalization on a limited basis through crying and cooing. Nursing strategies appropriate for children at this stage include the use of touch; speaking in a high pitched, gentle voice; maintaining eye contact with the infant; and using play appropriately (e.g., "peekaboo"). The older infant, age 6 to 12 months, builds on what has been learned previously. At this age, the infant is starting to become egocentric (the child sees him- or herself as the center of the universe). The infant begins to build a vocabulary with the first words spoken at 6 to 7 months of age. At this stage, the infant begins to experience "stranger anxiety" (a new behavior that involves with-

drawing from or rejecting unfamiliar people) and has no sense of object permanence (when an object is out of sight, it does not exist). Nursing strategies on which to focus include all that were used with the younger infant; in addition, the nurse should look for clues that the infant wants to play or interact, as through eye contact or reaching out with his or her arms.[1]

The toddler/preschool years span a large range, from 1 to 6 years of age. These children remain egocentric and focus on communication for and about themselves, how they feel, and what they can do. Toddlers continue to communicate with their hands when the words are not there. Toddlers and preschoolers rapidly acquire language skills, including rapid growth in vocabulary and in the ability to use it in sentences as they reach the preschool years. At this age, the child easily misinterprets phrases and interprets words literally. For example, "coughing your head off" means that your head will fall off of your body; "a little stick in the arm" means a tree stick will be put in the child's arm; and "bleeding out" means blood will come out of the body without stopping. The child is a concrete thinker at this age.

Communication strategies for toddlers include using patience in listening because it sometimes takes the child extra time to express his or her thoughts in words. Do not interrupt the child. Do not discuss frightening or serious subjects with the parents in the presence of the child. Choose your words carefully, keeping in mind the possibility of misinterpretations. Set limits for the child to provide a sense of security. Offer structured choices and redirect and/or reframe behavior when warranted. For example, the child can be given a choice between two different foods for lunch rather than asking an open-ended question such as, "What would you like to eat for lunch?" Using play as a form of communication can enhance the child's ability to tell you what is needed or desired. Age-appropriate play is discussed in greater detail later in this chapter.

The school-age period includes children ages 6 to 12. The child in this age group wants explanations and reasons for everything, such as what procedures are being done to him or her step-by-step and why. The school-age child is an enthusiastic participant in communication who needs relatively simple explanations at the beginning of the stage of development. As the child progresses from thinking concretely early in this age period to more abstract thinking as the end of this period approaches, more complete explanations can be given. A child at this age wants to use logic and often misinterprets adult conversations. Nursing strategies to focus on include using simple, straightforward questions and answers. The school-age child is often reluctant to communicate his or her own needs, so speaking and responding in the third person is useful in communication. For example, the nurse remarks, "Some children like to hold my hand when their IV is started." It is also important for the nurse to obtain the child's perceptions before any explanations are given to avoid confusion.

The adolescent period ranges from 12 to 18 years in age. This child fluctuates between childlike and adult thinking and behavior. The adolescent has a genuine interest in the care that is being provided and wants to participate in the decision-making process. As the later teen years approach, the adolescent is caught between wanting to be "grown up" and the security that comes from remaining a child. The adolescent has attitudes and feelings that need to be communicated about a wide range of topics from peer groups to identity, sex, substance abuse, and his or her parents. The nurse must recognize where and when to discuss these issues with the adolescent and how much communication can take place with and without the parents. Communicating with the adolescent begins with the development of trust. It is essential for the nurse to build a rapport with the adolescent, to listen vs talk, and to be nonjudgmental and straightforward. Although you may not approve of some of the adolescent's behavior, it is important to communicate acceptance of the person. The nurse must let the adolescent control the communication within the limitations of confidentiality without minimizing thoughts and feelings.[1,3]

■ COMMUNICATION STRATEGIES WITH CHILDREN

There are many traditional as well as nontraditional communication techniques that can be very successful with children of all ages. These communication techniques can be delineated as being either verbal, nonverbal, or a combination of both. Verbal techniques include word games and storytelling. Nonverbal techniques include drawing and story writing. For example, to learn more about the child's family relationships, you could ask the child to draw a picture of him- or herself and family members doing an activity together. Then ask the child to tell you about the drawing. This strategy engages the child in talking about how he or she views his or her family. Combination communication techniques center on various forms of play therapy. Young children will often spontaneously act out their experiences with dolls or plush animals and reveal their feelings and concerns. Communicating with children takes time and patience, thought and skill, creativity and practice, and, of course, a desire to communicate with children in whatever way possible to reach each unique individual.

The following list of "do's" and "don'ts" were adapted from Boggs'[4] recommendations for establishing rapport with children.

Table 7-1   Tips for Effective Communication with Children

Do	Do not
Get to know a child's developmental level	Make a child self-conscious by drawing attention to him or her
Learn the child's interests based on your observations of his or her activities	Use abstractions with a child who is a concrete thinker (e.g., for a child who does not understand time, tell him or her "after lunch," not "later" or "at 2 o'clock")
Talk at the child's level and with vocabulary he or she will understand	
"Level the playing field" by sharing your thoughts and/or observations about what is happening to the child	Jump to conclusions
Maintain a calm, unhurried, caring, gentle approach	Get "in the middle" between a child and a parent, especially in front of the child
Use concrete examples and/or link information to activities of daily living vs abstractions	
Allow opinions to be expressed	
Be an active, attentive listener	

Source: Adapted from Boggs, K. (2005). Communicating with children. In E. Arnold, K. Boggs, Eds. *Interpersonal Relationships: Professional Communication Skills for Nurses* (5th ed.). Philadelphia: WB Saunders.

Sydnor-Greenberg and Dokken[5] conducted a study of communication patterns between children and health care providers. They interviewed children ages 4 to 17 and then interviewed the children's mothers separately. Based on their interviews, the researchers developed the "CLEAR" communication framework: "C" is the context of the communication between the child and the health care provider. The child is more than just a diagnosis or health problem. He or she has a life outside of the illness and wants that to be acknowledged by the health care provider. "L" is for listening to the child, actively listening to what he or she has to say, what he or she does not say, and what he or she needs help saying. Listening is a partnership that requires participation by both the child and the health care provider. "E" is for empowerment. Empowerment implies an active role for the child. Children want to know, to be informed, and to have meaningful input to any communication. Children do not want to be talked about, overlooked, ignored, or "brushed off," as if to say their input is irrelevant and not necessary. "A" stands for advice, providing relevant information to the child. Children want to be taught and want to know what lies ahead and how they can assist in the management of their care. This data allows the child a certain degree of independence, which he or she would be working toward if he or she were outside the health care environment. "R" stands for reassurance that the child is recovering, healthy, and managing his or her care well. Children do not want false reassurance any more than adults do; children don't want to be lied to, nor do they want the truth to be omitted completely.

■ CHILD-SPECIFIC COMMUNICATION STRATEGIES

The following strategies can be used to better assess the child and to give him or her an opportunity to express any needs.

Word Games

Word games are an effective means of communicating, especially for children who have at least a moderate degree of language development. Word games can include a version of the "happy faces" game in which the nurse asks the child to describe how his or her face looks today, yesterday, and how it will look tomorrow. The nurse should focus on the words the child uses. Do the words change with the child's perception of health, and are the words more positive or negative in tone? Word games can be extended to word association, moving from more neutral words to more anxiety-provoking words. "Describe in one word how you feel." "Sick," "surgery," "hospital," and other words that are specific to the health/illness experience can be used. The nurse needs to remember that word games must be appropriate for the child's age and cognitive and developmental stages.

Storytelling

Storytelling can be guided and/or directed, as in "tell a story about a girl/boy like you," or "tell a story about this picture." Storytelling can also be free, as in "tell about anything you want." Storytelling allows reality and imagination to become integrated. By creating characters in a story, children can express concerns and explore what is happening to them without becoming too personally invested. Storytelling allows the child to communicate in a comfortable way with control over the communication process. The more focused the nurse wants the child to be, the more guidance or direction should be given. The more exploration the nurse wants the child to do, the less guidance and direction the nurse should give. It is important to stress that too much structure can shift the child's communication. The nurse needs to allow the child to dictate the direction of the story. The child needs to be able to be creative, imaginative, and real according to his or her own ability, and the nurse must then extrapolate the meaning of the story based on clues the child is giving/communicating.

Drawing

Drawing is another means of encouraging a child to express him- or herself without words. It allows the externalization of internal mental images and emotions.[6] Depending on age, drawing is an activity that children often do in the normal course of a day; therefore, it is safe and familiar. When using drawing as a communication technique, the emphasis is not on how well the picture is drawn but in the ability to get in touch with feelings and healing through the drawing. When a child is not verbally sophisticated, drawing can be extremely helpful in facilitating communication. When a child is overwhelmed by experiences, the environment, or the uncertain or unknown, drawing can be therapeutic. The nurse can gain insight into a child who is undergoing painful procedures or experiencing fears, concerns, or problems through the process of drawing.

Drawing can be structured in that the child can be asked to draw something specific about an emotion or experience. Unstructured drawing or asking a child to draw whatever he or she wants is a very effective method to explore feelings and concerns. The child can be encouraged to include written details of the drawn images if he or she so desires. Drawings can be in black and white or include colors. Let the child decide which colors to use because color is expressive of emotions. There are toys available to allow the child to use colors to express themselves such as a color wand or color changing necklace[7] to express mood in color. Drawings can include symbols as well, again to be determined by the child rather than the nurse. Drawing as a form of communication can be very effective in facilitating expression of a child's deepest emotions. DiGallo, Netzer-Stein, and Winkler[8] found that drawing allowed children with cancer to express their fears and could also be used to assess a child's ability to cope.

Story Writing

Story writing is similar to storytelling but is used with an older child or adolescent. Story writing can be used to express or communicate feelings, thoughts, beliefs, and/or fears that can be verbally expressed. The writing process can take many forms, from actual event-driven stories to journal writing, writing letters to an actual person or to oneself, or writing on the Internet. The Internet offers several possibilities including e-mail, chat rooms, or by posting a story on a Web page. Story writing can be cathartic or an emotional release. Writing allows personal reflection while maintaining some degree of privacy. Story writing, like storytelling, can be both structured and unstructured. The nurse can be guided by clues from the child as to which actually will accomplish the therapeutic goal most effectively.

Play

Play is children's work. It is what they know, what they understand, and it is how they communicate. In play, children utilize both verbal and nonverbal communication skills to express their feelings without acknowledging cognitively and/or intellectually that they are doing so. Play can be structured or free and can take on many forms depending on the age and cognitive development of the child. Play activities as a form of communication can include simple hand games with an infant, "peekaboo" with an older infant, play with safe medical equipment for the older toddler and preschooler, doll play, and more technical medical play with the school-age child. Older children may enjoy activities on the computer such as participating in an online support group or sending e-mail to the nurse. For the more sophisticated play of the adolescent, include more advanced computer activities such as creating a Web page to tell their story and sharing it with others such as the nurse or other adolescents experiencing a similar problem. All of these play activities serve as a means of safe, acceptable communication between the child and the nurse.

Imaginary Friends

Imaginary friends are a form of play therapy that is often utilized by older preschoolers and school-age children. Their desire to communicate in the third person makes the use of an imaginary friend acceptable to them and an avenue from which they can communicate about themselves without acknowledging the connection. Imaginary friends "arrive" for a reason and should not be ignored or criticized. Imaginary friends serve a purpose for children. Children talk to the "friend"; they allow their friend to talk for them, expressing how they feel, while maintaining their own inner self. Nurses and parents need to acknowledge the friend and allow this "friendship" to run its course. When the child no longer needs an imaginary friend, the friend will go away.

■ CHILDREN WITH NONTRADITIONAL COMMUNICATION PATTERNS

Impaired communication in children included the "inability to 1) receive or process symbol systems for the spoken word; 2) to represent concepts or symbol systems; or 3) transmit and use symbol systems"[9] (p. 1017). A communication impairment may occur in speech (expression of thoughts in words), hearing, language (the cognitive process by which speech is created and understood), or any combination of these three components. Delayed language and speech development is often found in children with developmental delays. Speech problems are more common than language problems, but both can improve with age.[9]

Autism is a complex developmental disorder of brain function. Autism is accompanied by a broad range

Case example

When verbal communication is uncomfortable for a child, for whatever reason, play activities can assist the child in communicating his or her feelings. The following clinical case study illustrates the very important connection between play and communication with a child.

Mark is a 10-year-old boy who was admitted to the hospital with a diagnosis of vesicoureteral reflux and who was scheduled for a surgical repair. Following surgery, Mark had a Foley catheter in place that was to be advanced daily by the urologist. Each morning, the nurse noticed that as the time grew closer to the doctor arriving, Mark's vital signs increased, and he became agitated and diaphoretic. When asked what was wrong or if he wanted to talk, he closed his eyes and pulled the covers up to his chin. One day, the nurse stayed with him as he heard the footsteps of the doctor down the hall. His increased anxiety was consistent with the anticipation of what was to occur—the advancement of his catheter.

Based on the clues Mark had given, the nurse had an idea about an age/developmentally appropriate means of communication that would possibly encourage him to deal with his feelings about the threatening situation he was experiencing. The nurse took a pillowcase and stuffed it with filling then tied it at the end. She took it to Mark with a big black marker and told him the pillow was his to do with as he wished. He drew the face of the doctor on it and he even put the doctor's name on top. The nurse put a hook through the top and connected it to the patient drape rod that encircled the room. She placed the "doc" in front of Mark and left him alone for a few minutes. She watched from the hallway as Mark punched it. As he hit it, it went all around the room on the rod on the ceiling and came back in front of him. What a smile Mark had as he continued this anxiety-relieving activity! The next day, when he heard the doctor's footsteps, he asked the nurse for the "punching bag," and he went at it. He was communicating his feelings through play with both his illustration on the bag and his actions with the bag. Every day for the next 4 days, Mark performed the same activity prior to the doctor arriving. During this period he was calmer, his vital signs remained stable, and he was in control. When Mark was finally discharged, he asked to take his "punching bag" home with him. He even asked the doctor to sign it, which he did. Play, the ultimate communication technique of children, was very effective in this case.

of intellectual and behavioral deficits, among them are speech and language delays. A child with autism may demonstrate difficulty communicating ranging from the inability to make eye contact to a total lack of speech and language. The American Psychological Association[10] outlines diagnostic criteria for autism that relate to communication:

1) delay in, or total lack of, the development of spoken language, not accompanied by an attempt to compensate through alternative modes of communication such as gesture or mime;

2) in children with adequate speech, marked impairment in the ability to initiate or sustain a conversation with others;

3) stereotyped and repetitive use of language or idiosyncratic language; and

4) lack of varied, spontaneous make-believe play or social initiative play appropriate to developmental level. (p. 75)

The American Academy of Neurology[11] recommends evaluation of any child who does not display language skills, such as babbling or gesturing, by 12 months of age, no single word by 16 months of age, and a lack of two word phrases by 24 months of age.

Attention deficit hyperactivity disorder (ADHD) is characterized by abnormally high levels of inattention, impulsiveness, and hyperactivity in relation to a child's developmental level.[9] The most prominent symptom is distractibility. The cause of distractibility may be internal or may come from external sources. In addition to distractibility, other symptoms include immaturity relative to a child's chronological age and excessive risk taking, particularly physical risk taking.[1,12] Distractibility will influence the child's ability to attend and respond to communication. Inattentiveness may result in lack of social participation by the child, inappropriate comments, or lack of congruence between the theme of a conversation and a child's contributions to the conversation.

■ STRATEGIES TO ENHANCE COMMUNICATION WHEN CHILDREN USE NONTRADITIONAL COMMUNICATION PATTERNS

Overall, the primary intervention for communication disorders is prevention whenever possible. Prevention strategies directly relate to factors that may predispose causes of language/speech impairment, including hearing loss. Early recognition and appropriate referrals are essential to the promotion of adequate language development and communication skills.[9]

Strategies to improve communication techniques specifically for children with autism revolve around the use of highly structured and intensive behavioral modification programs. It is critical for health care providers, as well as family members, to present an atmosphere where positive reinforcement is promoted. There must be an effort to provide the child with opportunities for increasing social awareness of others, opportunities for teaching verbal communication skills, in addition to decreasing unacceptable behavior.[9] The key to facilitating communication in an autistic child is to provide opportunities for interaction in a routine, structured environment.

Parents and teachers must convey consistent messages to the child. The more structured the environment, the easier it is to communicate consistently, thus the more successful the child can be. Examples of structured communication include written communication such as lists of activities, homework assignments, tasks at home, and daily schedules.

A child with ADHD will have difficulty receiving messages as well as transmitting them. Medications can help decrease distractibility. Most children with ADHD are treated with methylphenidate (Ritalin) or dexamfetaminesulphate.[13] Methylphenidate causes an increase in dopamine and norepinephrine levels, stimulating the inhibitory system of the central nervous system. To get maximum benefit as it relates to the child's need to function and communicate in school, the medication is usually given with breakfast and at lunchtime.

Beyond the traditional pharmacological interventions for the treatment of ADHD, there are other key strategies to ensure successful childhood development, including effective communication. A multidisciplinary approach must be utilized, including behavioral strategies and/or psychotherapy, environmental manipulation, and appropriate classroom placement.[12] Because a child with ADHD is often in school, it is critical to include the teacher as well as the school nurse in any and all interventions related to the child and his or her communication in this learning environment.

The teacher, as well as the parents, must be sure to minimize distractions in the environment, provide a consistent study/work area, and provide predictability in daily scheduling to enhance the child's communication successes. Additionally, giving the child both verbal and written instructions and scheduling more difficult tasks in the morning, when the medications are at their peak blood levels, will increase the child's potential for success.

■ CONCLUSION

Communication with children is not defined by a script, by generalities, or by steadfast rules. Communication with children is dictated by each child's unique characteristics, including his or her age, cognitive development, language development, experiences, and the child's ability to express him- or herself through both verbal and nonverbal means. A child's ability to communicate changes and evolves over time. Nurses must be aware that communicating with a child involves appreciating the uniqueness of that child, having a general understanding of the physical and psychosocial development of children, having the patience to allow the child to express him- or herself using a variety of traditional and nontraditional methods, and being flexible. Two guiding principles are 1) no two children are alike; and 2) children are not miniature adults. To communicate with children effectively, the nurse must see the world through their eyes.

REFERENCES

1. Hockenberry, M. (2003). *Wong's nursing care of infants and children.* St. Louis, MO: CV Mosby.

2. Chitty, K. (2005). *Professional nursing: Concepts and challenges.* St. Louis, MO: WB Saunders.

3. Deering, C., & Cody, D. (2002). Communicating with children and adolescents. *American Journal of Nursing, 102*(3), 34–41.

4. Boggs, K. (2005). Communicating with children. In E. Arnold & K. Boggs (Eds.), *Interpersonal relationships: Professional communication skills for nurses* (5th ed.). Philadelphia: WB Saunders.

5. Sydnor-Greenberg, N., & Dokken, D. (2001). Communication in healthcare: Thoughts on the child's perception. *Journal of Child and Family Nursing, 4*(3), 225–230.

6. Dossey, B., Keegan, L., Guzzetta, C., & Kolkmeier, L. (2005). *Holistic nursing: A handbook for practice.* Gaithersburg, MD: Aspen Publishing.

7. Funkytownhall.com. Retrieved March 22, 2007, from http://www.funkytownmall.com/product_info.php?products_id=666981

8. DiGallo, A., Netzer-Stein, A., & Winkler, R. (2001). Drawing as a means of communication at the initial interview with children with cancer. *Journal of Child Psychotherapy, 27*(2), 197–210.

9. Hockenberry, M. (2003). *Wong's nursing care of infants and children.* St. Louis, MO: CV Mosby.

10. American Psychiatric Association. (2000). *Diagnostic and statistical manual of mental disorders (DSM-IV-TR).* Washington, DC: American Psychiatric Association.

11. Filipek, P.A. (2000). Practice parameter: Screening and diagnosis of autism. Report of the Quality Standards Subcommittee of the American Academy of Neurology and the Child Neurology Society. *Neurology, 55*(2), 468–479.

12. Law, S., & Schachar, R. (1999). Do typical clinical doses of methylphenidate cause tics in children treated for attention deficit hyperactivity disorder? *Journal of American Academy of Child and Adolescent Psychiatry, 38*(8), 944–951.

13. King, S., Griffin, S., Hodges, Z., Weatherby, H., Ausseburg, C., Richardson, G., et al. (2006). A systematic review and economic model of the effectiveness and cost-effectiveness of methylphenidate, dexamfetamine, and atomoxetine for the treatment of attention deficit hyperactivity disorder in children and adolescents. *Health Technology Assessment, 10*(23), iii–iv, xiii–146.

EXERCISES

1. Self-Assessment

Working with children is both exciting and challenging. Seeing the world through their eyes takes some imagination. It may help you recall your own childhood experiences with illness. Imagine a time when you were a child and you were ill, required surgery, or you were hospitalized. In your self-assessment notebook, communicate this experience either through a writing exercise (story, poem, narrative) or by drawing a picture depicting what that experience was like for you. Spend 5 to 10 minutes sharing those experiences with a confidant.

2. Responding to Situations

A. Suzy, an 11-year-old, is admitted to your unit for corrective surgery for scoliosis. You must complete preoperative teaching with her. Based on her age and cognitive level (she is age appropriate), what is the best communication technique to utilize with Suzy and why? Specifically, develop age- and cognitively appropriate teaching strategies to teach Suzy what she should expect.

B. Interpret the following (in writing) from the point of view of a toddler:

1. "It will feel like a mosquito bite."

2. "It is just a quick stick in your leg."

3. "You are just going to have your cast cut off."

4. "You sound like you are going to cough your head off."

5. "I need to take some blood from you."

C. Now develop age-specific methods for communicating these ideas to toddlers using words or other appropriate methods.

    1. "It will feel like a mosquito bite."

    2. "It is just a quick stick in your leg."

    3. "You are just going to have your cast cut off."

    4. "You sound like you are going to cough your head off."

    5. "I need to take some blood from you."

8

Communicating with Older Adults

Theris A. Touhy DNP, APRN, BC and Christine L. Williams, DNSc, APRN, BC

Touch the gnarled hand. Smooth the wispy, thin hair back from the lined face. Offer a cool drink to the parched lips. Caress lotion onto the frail skin. Speak to the speechless. Hear the cries. Hear the silence. Slip into the darkened room. Be present. Do not fear that there may be no purpose. Do not be afraid to face who you or someone you love may one day become. There is much to be learned. Do not let another's pain dampen and drown your soul, and turn you away. Allow yourself to learn from those whom you think you cannot learn from. Let them step into your very being. Learn what they have to teach. Learn even if they cannot speak, even if it seems they cannot respond at all. Listen to the beating of your heart. Open the shadows of your mind. Be present.[1]

OBJECTIVES

1. To consider the significance of communication in the lives of older adults

2. To discuss the detrimental effects of ageism on communication with older clients

3. To explore strategies to improve communication with older adults

4. To describe communication challenges common to older clients and adaptations to meet those challenges

■ COMMUNICATION WITH ELDERS

The ability to communicate and engage with others in meaningful interactions is fundamental to quality of life and well-being for all people. The need to communicate, to be listened to, and to feel that one's words and messages are valued and respected does not change with age or impairment.[2] In fact, social contact is vital to older adults' emotional and physical well being.[3] Social interaction improves older adults' chances of living longer and maintaining optimal functional abilities.[4] Sadly, older people are at risk for isolation and may find fewer opportunities for social interaction. The death of friends and relatives, illnesses, and other losses such as moving out of one's home and relocating to smaller apartments, assisted living, or nursing homes may decrease access to social support from others.[5] Communication between nurses and older people tends to be superficial or task focused.[6,7]

This chapter focuses on special considerations for therapeutic communication with older adults, the effects of ageism, speech and language disorders, and sensory impairment on therapeutic communication with older people, and it presents nursing responses to enhance communication and mutual caring.

■ AGEISM AND COMMUNICATION

Therapeutic communication techniques that apply to all nursing situations, such as authentic presence, mutuality, active listening, clarifying, giving information, seeking validation of understanding, keeping focus, and using open-ended questions, are applicable in communicating with older adults.[2] Unfortunately, ageist attitudes often influence formal caregivers (nurses, nursing students, residential staff) and even family members to communicate in ways that demean rather than demonstrate respect for the autonomy of older people.[8] Ageism may be displayed when health care providers use "elderspeak" to communicate with older adults. Elderspeak is a form of speech that is overly nurturing, patronizing, controlling, and disrespectful.[9] Based on a faulty assumption that all elders will have difficulty comprehending speech, younger people alter their speech patterns by slowing the pace of speech, using a louder, high pitched tone (similar to baby talk), and simplifying the message.[10] Overly nurturing and patronizing talk is used to control.[11] The use of pet names or diminutives is one way that the caregiver can imply an inappropriately intimate, patronizing, or even parent–child relationship. Collective pronouns such as "we" imply that the elder is not autonomous. Tag questions are also controlling because they suggest the answer for the elder. The following example illustrates several features of elderspeak.

> Mrs. Blanco is an 85-year-old Hispanic woman who is recovering from a stroke. At 7 a.m., the nurse greets her using elderspeak: "Come on now Mamma, we need to sit you up so that you can have your medicine. Come on, you wouldn't want to spill this, would you?"

In the prior example, "Mamma" is a pet name, also known as a diminutive. The use of diminutives such as "sweetie," "honey," "grandma," or use of a first name without the client's permission implies inequality in the relationship, control by the nurse, and communicates disrespect for the elder. Many older people are not used to our informal styles of communicating, so ask them how they would like to be addressed. It is always desirable to use Mr., Miss, or Mrs. until you are told otherwise.

In the phrase "we need you to sit up," "we" is a collective pronoun that communicates expectations of incompetence or a client's inability to act without the nurse. Tag questions that include both the question and the answer are another strategy to decrease the client's autonomy ("you wouldn't want to spill this, would you?"). Giving control to the elder is communicated by knocking on a door, introducing yourself clearly, and asking permission to enter or providing some choice by asking, "Are you ready to walk now?"[12]

Other forms of communication that convey ageist attitudes include ignoring the older person while communicating with relatives or visitors or limiting interaction to task-focused communication. Be sure to speak directly to the elder and involve him or her in all conversations. If family or significant others are present, they may be asked for their input as appropriate, but the focus of the communication is on the elder. It is important that others not answer for elders or talk about them as if they were not present. If it is important to validate information, this can be done privately with the family or significant other. This is true when working with both cognitively intact and cognitively impaired elders.

While an understanding of basic therapeutic communication skills and adaptations for age is important, the nurse must realize that the most important communication tool they possess is the use of self. The unique contribution that nursing brings to the care of people is the intimate, knowing of the person behind the disease and the creation of relationships and interactions that support, validate, and celebrate the person as someone of value and worth.[13] Every time a nurse communicates with someone, their words and actions affect the relationship in either positive or negative ways depending on their attitude and skills.[14] Relating to the person being nursed as a fellow human being and truly reaching out on a more intimate and caring level, rather than in a rote manner, will foster the development of healing relationships. When caring for elders in a busy setting such as a hospital, it is easy for nurses to overlook the social interactions that are part of optimal relationships. Although it may consume a little more time, the importance of greeting the elder and orienting him or her to what you are doing cannot be overstated (e.g., "I'm here to talk about your discharge plans."). Ageist attitudes and fear of our own aging often direct our communication with older people. These factors may blind our eyes to seeing the person behind the disease or impairment and prevent us from entering into caring relationships that enrich the lives of both the nurse and the person being nursed.

■ SPECIAL CONSIDERATIONS FOR COMMUNICATING WITH ELDERS

Because older people have a larger life experience to draw from, they may need more time to answer questions or provide information. Sorting through thoughts may require intervals of silence, and word retrieval may be slower for older people. "Older people use fewer proper nouns, more general nouns, and more ambiguous references as they age" (p. 95).[15] Avoid hurrying older patients and try to give them a few extra minutes to talk about their concerns or express their feelings. Listen attentively and patiently, not interrupting the person. If you tend to speak quickly, especially if your accent differs from the elder's, try to slow down further and give the older person time to process what you are saying.[16] Repeating or rephrasing questions, asking for clarification, and frequently seeking validation of what you think you heard are other techniques that facilitate communication. Pay attention to the client's gaze, gestures, body language, and the pitch, volume, and tone of the patient's voice to help you understand what the person is trying to communicate. Both eye contact and physical touch communicate caring from the nurse and can aid in understanding and being understood without words. Sundin and Jansson describe eye contact as "looking through soft eyes and seeing the person with the heart" (p. 114).[17]

Open-ended questions may be difficult for some elders. The older person may try to respond with what they think you would like to hear rather than what it is they would like to say. Some elders fear "being a bother" or may be concerned about taking up too much of your time. When using closed questioning to obtain specific information, the elder may feel pressured, and the appropriate information may not be immediately forthcoming. Older people may also be hesitant to provide information for fear of the consequences. An example might be a question related to falls. If the person lives alone and has been falling in their own home, sharing that information may mean that they have to move to a more protective setting.

Assessment questions can be anxiety producing situations for elders. Older people may not be able to answer correctly because of fear and nervousness, or they may feel threatened if questions are asked in a quizzing or demanding manner. It's often helpful to begin an assessment by saying something like: "I am going to ask you some questions. Just relax and try to answer the best that you can." It is important to create an environment of acceptance, support, and caring and to put the elder in the best situation for meaningful communication. This may mean communicating at their best time of day or when they are rested as well as communicating in a quiet and private environment with minimal distractions. Starting the conversation with casual topics (weather, special interests) before beginning a detailed assessment may put the person at ease. Asking them to share their major concerns first, regardless of the priority of the nursing assessment, is also important.

Memories are important to elders, and some may want to talk about their past and share their memories with you. Careful listening to stories and reminiscence is a more complete way to enter into their life and come to know the person. Older people bring us complex stories that are derived from many years of living. To enter into the world of an elder and come to know them in their wholeness requires time and patience and a belief that the story and the person are valuable and meaningful. The metaphor of an old house can be used to illuminate knowing wholeness of older adults. When you think of an older adult, picture a house with many rooms, doors, and windows. Life stories are revealed slowly and only after trust has been established. It may take a long time for you to be invited in to see all of the rooms. If you remain on the front porch or sit only in the formal living room, the story you hear may be very different from the one you hear when you are invited to share the treasures and memories of the rest of the house.[18]

Stories serve as a mirror in that they image those life events most dear to the storyteller, and the language of stories helps us uncover that which makes life meaningful. Sandelowski describes story as a narrative knowing, which is essential knowing for providers of health care. Stories are "critical sources of information about etiology, diagnosis, treatment, and prognosis from the patient's point of view" (p. 25).[19] Without this knowing, older people are subject to less than accurate diagnoses, labels that reflect ageist attitudes, and treatment that focuses on incomplete knowing. With no knowledge of the person's story, how can we begin to extend our care, to understand behavior, to diagnose and treat concerns, and to design responses that nurture wholeness? As Coles states, "the people who come to see us bring us their stories. They hope that we tell them well enough so that we understand the truth of their lives. They hope we understand how to interpret their stories correctly" (p. 7).[20] When nurses take the time to listen to older people share memories and life stories, they communicate respect and valuing of the individual and his or her life as something very important to be treasured.

Both the nurse and the person being nursed grow as a result of interactions grounded in respect and valuing.

■ COMMUNICATING WHEN CLIENTS HAVE SENSORY DEFICITS

Elders may have sensory impairments that put them more at risk for experiencing communication difficulties than people of younger ages. This may be especially true for frail elders such as those in nursing homes where it is estimated that "nearly half of the residents never talk to other residents because of hearing and speech difficulties" (p. 96).[15] Communication with older people who have sensory deficits requires special skills. Nurses may not recognize sensory impairments or appreciate their impact on the individual's functioning, or they may view sensory impairments as obstacles to communication and limit communication with older people. Assume that the person can hear, see, or understand you unless you know in advance that this is not the case.[8]

Vision and Vision Impairment

As they age, all people are affected by presbyopia. Presbyopia is the condition of vision in which the normally flexible lens of the eye gradually loses elasticity, affecting the refractive ability of the eye. Presbyopia affects the ability of the eyes to accommodate close and detailed work. Usually it is noticed when one has difficulty reading close up and begins holding reading materials farther away. It affects everyone, and there is no known prevention. Presbyopia begins in the fourth decade and continues throughout the rest of one's life. Nearly everyone over 45 years old requires glasses for close vision. Presbyopia occurs earlier in individuals who live in warm climates where there is a lot of sun exposure and later in individuals who are nearsighted (myopia).

Other normal age-related changes in vision include a decrease in pupil size and a slower response of the pupil to light. These changes cause problems with adaptation to darkness and when moving from one light level to another (e.g., entering a dark theater from a brightly lit lobby). Night vision decreases and many older people avoid driving at night. Glare is also a major problem that is created not only by sunlight outdoors but also by the reflection of light on any shiny object, such as light striking a highly polished floor (often seen in hospitals and nursing homes).[2] As a result of pupil changes and a reduced translucency of the cornea, lens, and vitreous humor, older people require three times the amount of light to see things as they did when they were in their 20s. Adequate lighting is important, and it is more effective to use high-intensity lighting focused on the object or surface than to increase the overall lighting of the room. Increasing lens opacity and the development of cataracts affects color clarity. Warmer and more intense colors, such as red and orange, are more easily seen than blue or green or beige. This is important in designing environments as well as teaching materials.

According to the Centers for Disease Control and Prevention, 1.8 million community-dwelling elders report difficulty with activities of daily living because of visual impairment, and 2.7 million older people have severe visual impairment. Among nursing home residents, estimates of visual impairment range from 21% to 52%.[21] Visual impairment affects not only communication but also functional ability, safety, and quality of life. Visual impairment is considered to be vision loss that cannot be corrected by glasses or contact lenses. Snellen wall chart readings of 20/40 or worse with corrective lenses is considered to be visual impairment, and Snellen readings of 20/200 or more are considered to be legal blindness or severe visual impairment. Racial disparities exist with African Americans being twice as likely to be visually impaired as whites of comparable socioeconomic status. The major causes of visual impairment and blindness among older adults are cataracts, macular degeneration, glaucoma, and diabetic retinopathy. It is important to note that many of these visual impairments can be diagnosed early with appropriate eye care, but many older people, particularly ethnically and racially diverse elders, do not receive necessary care.

Communicating with Elders with Visual Impairment

Social interaction includes both verbal and nonverbal communication. In fact, most communication is nonverbal. For visually impaired elders to participate optimally in the communication process, it is important to facilitate visualization of the speaker's face whenever possible. Assist the elder to wear eyeglasses and be sure that they are clean. Eyeglasses are often misplaced in transfers between homes and institutions, so be sure to find out if the elder has glasses and obtain them. Provide adequate lighting so that the elder can see your facial expressions and read your lips. Don't obstruct the elder's view by covering your mouth or chewing during conversation. Other strategies are found in Table 8-1.

Hearing and Hearing Impairment

Hearing impairment affects more than one third of community-dwelling elders and an estimated 90% of nursing home residents. Older men are more likely than older women to be hearing impaired.[16,22] Like vision impairment, hearing impairment affects functional ability and quality of life. Hearing loss contributes to miscommunication, misdiagnosis, medication errors, functional decline, social isolation, depression, and even paranoia.[22,23] Impaired hearing increases isolation and suspicion and can lead to paranoid behavior. Because older people with a hearing loss may not understand or respond appropriately to a conversation, they may be labeled as confused or cognitively impaired. Research suggests that assessment, recognition, and management of hearing loss is not adequate in health care. Nurses play an important role in identifying hearing impairment in their patients and providing strategies to enhance communication.

The two major forms of hearing loss are conductive and sensorineural. Conductive hearing loss involves abnormalities of the external and middle ear such as otosclerosis, perforated eardrum, fluid in the middle ear, or cerumen accumulation (often overlooked but easy to resolve). Sensorineural hearing loss is caused by damage to any part of the inner ear or neural pathways to the brain. Systemic disease, noise exposure, ototoxic substances, and some medications can cause this type of hearing loss.[22] Presbycusis is a type of sensorineural hearing loss that affects people over the age of 50 and is the most common cause of hearing loss in the United States. Presbycusis is a bilateral hearing loss associated with loss of the ability to distinguish high-pitched sounds. Consonants used in speech such as *s, sh, t,* and *p* are high frequency sounds while vowels are low-frequency sounds. Consonants help make speech distinct and understandable, and the inability to hear these sounds makes language disjointed and misunderstood. The common reaction of raising one's voice or shouting to communicate with people who have presbycusis compounds this problem because high-pitched sounds drop out of speech when the voice is raised.[23]

Presbycusis occurs gradually, and people may be initially unaware of their loss of hearing, often blaming others for mumbling or slurring their words. Older people may also be sensitive to admitting hearing loss. It is

Table 8-1   Strategies for Communicating with Elders Who Have Impaired Vision

Do	Do not
• Get down to the person's level	• Startle the elder by touching without warning
• Face the person	• Cover your mouth with your hand
• Increase intensity of lighting	• Eat, chew gum
• Ensure adequate lighting for your face	• Exaggerate pronunciation
• Eliminate glare	• Speak quickly and change topics rapidly
• Use nonverbal approaches; supportive touch	• Assume the person cannot understand you if they have vision problems
• Eliminate physical barriers such as a table or a desk	• Stand at the door of the room or at the bedside above the patient and look down to communicate
• Use the analogy of a clock face to help locate objects such as food on a plate	
• Do not change the room arrangement or move personal items without explanation	
• Select colors with good intensity (red, orange)	
• Use large, dark, evenly spaced printing	
• Use contrast in printed material (e.g., black on white, not beige on beige)	
• Be aware of low-vision assistive devices that may be helpful for the person (talking clocks and watches, talking books) and connect them to these resources	

important to establish rapport with the person and open with a comment such as: "Many people have hearing difficulty in certain situations. Have you experienced any difficulty? Can you tell me about it?" The Hearing Handicap Inventory (HHIE-S) is a quick screening tool.[22] Other symptoms of hearing impairment include repeated requests to speak louder, leaning forward or cupping the hand over the ear during conversations, difficulty hearing on the telephone, inappropriate responses or inattention during conversations, and difficulty hearing the voices of women or children (more high-pitched) or hearing in noisy areas.[22] An inability to filter out background noises is also associated with presbycusis. Avoid communicating in noisy environments (restaurants, hospitals) or when the television is on to optimize hearing ability.

Although hearing aids have improved considerably, only 20% of older people with hearing impairment purchase and consistently wear them.[22] Older people with visual deficits, arthritic hands, or cognitive impairments may have difficulty with hearing aids. Another assistive listening device that is helpful is a "pocket talker," a small unit similar to a Walkman that has an amplifying microphone and headset or ear piece.[2,22] These are not expensive and should be available in institutions and ambulatory care settings. Certified sign language interpreters, telecommunication devices, and telecaptioning devices on televisions should also be available for hearing impaired patients.

Hearing aids do not restore normal hearing but generally improve hearing by about 50%. Hearing aids should be fitted by trained professionals and require a period of training and adjustment. They are expensive, ranging in price from about $500 to several thousand dollars. It is very important that nurses know how the hearing aid works, how to put the aid in the ear of the person, and change the batteries. Like glasses, hearing aids often get misplaced during transfers or stays in institutions. Because they are lifelines to communication for people with hearing impairment, they should be treated with great care. The following story illustrates this point.

Communicating with Elders Who Have Hearing Impairment

It is important for the nurse to recognize and assess hearing impairment because it can adversely affect not only communication but also understanding and adherence to the medical regimen. Be alert to signs of hearing impair-

> Mr. Jackson was a 75-year-old man admitted to the extended care facility following a hospital stay for congestive heart failure. Whenever the staff attempted to provide physical care, he became very agitated, pushing them away and striking out. He appeared to be unable to understand any communication. A psychiatric consult was obtained, and he was diagnosed with dementia and placed on antipsychotic medications. About one week after he was admitted, his only living relative from out of town came to visit. He asked the staff what happened to his bilateral hearing aids and told them that he was "deaf as a post." Apparently his hearing aids had been lost during the hospital stay. Audiology was called, and he was given an assistive listening device while he was fitted for new hearing aids. When he was able to hear, it became clear that he had no cognitive impairment and was actually a very pleasant man who had been a nurse anesthetist.

ment such as inattention or inappropriate responses. If a person has been identified as having a hearing impairment, document it on the patient's record and communicate the information to all caregivers. Talk with the patient and family to determine the most effective way to communicate. Ensure that hearing aids, if used, are available and working and given proper care and storage to avoid loss. Inform the client of available resources to improve hearing. Augment conversation with gestures and visual aids. Other suggestions are presented in Table 8-2.

Communicating with Elders Who Have Speech and Language Impairments

Impairments in verbal communication can occur from neurological conditions such as head injury, stroke, Parkinson disease, and dementia. Aphasia may occur following a stroke and can affect speaking, understanding, reading, and writing. While communication changes due to hearing and vision impairments or dementia occur gradually, aphasia causes an instant impairment.[15] Depending on the area of the brain that is affected, aphasia may be fluent or nonfluent. People with fluent aphasia are able to speak easily, but the content does not make sense. People with fluent aphasia also have problems understanding spoken language and may be unaware of their difficulties. With nonfluent aphasia, speech is very limited or slow and the person has great difficulty articulating words. People with nonfluent aphasia usually understand others but may not be able to get out the words to respond. People with aphasia should be evaluated by a speech language pathologist. Speech rehabilitation programs can do much to improve communication as well as provide a plan of care to help the nurse communicate more effectively with the person who has aphasia. If speech cannot be improved, there are many assistive and augmentative communication devices that can be helpful, such as electronic boards, computers, and picture boards. The "Talking Mat" is a visual framework using picture symbols to aid in expression of feelings about activities, the environment, people in their lives, and their own personal interests and views. Research conducted with frail older people experiencing communication difficulty using a Talking Mat suggested that this is a valuable tool in enhancing communication and sharing of ideas and feelings.[15] Writing words or phrases that the person can point to when answering questions may also be helpful if his or her reading ability is not impaired.[24]

Attempts at communication can be very frustrating for both the person experiencing aphasia and the nurse who is trying to understand. In most cases, aphasia does not affect the intellectual ability of people, so it is important to treat them as adults. Avoid "talking down" or talking about them as if they were not there, explain all actions, and involve them in decisions. Encourage family members to do the same.

As stated in Boykin, Parker, and Touhy, "When the patient actively tries to communicate, the care provider stays silent. These moments of silence give the patient time to concentrate without disruption. Furthermore, the silence provides an increasing possibility for listening and comprehending with openness" (p. 112).[17]

The following describes how a nurse participant in a phenomenological study of care of patients with stroke and aphasia communicates.

When the patient does not understand what I am trying to do, I do not nag. I show him how

Table 8-2   Strategies for Communicating with Elders Who Have Impaired Hearing

Do	
Do	• Check the ears for cerumen impaction and, if present, arrange for removal
• Gain the person's attention before speaking	• Use assistive listening devices if appropriate
• Get down to the elder's eye level	• If the person uses sign language, try to avoid restrictions of arms and legs
• Face the older person when speaking	• Obtain a certified sign language interpreter if appropriate
• Eliminate background noise (turn off television, close door, consider eliminating noisy paging systems)	**Do not**
• Speak with normal volume	• Over enunciate
• Articulate clearly	• Raise your voice or shout
• Lower the pitch of your voice	• Speak in a high pitched voice
• Ask patient or family what helps the elder to hear best	• Communicate in noisy areas
• Orient the light on the speaker's face	• Communicate with the television or radio on
• Periodically verify comprehension to ensure understanding	• Cover your mouth
• Use normal pace	• Assume that the person cannot understand
• Use nonverbal approaches; gestures, demonstrations, visual aids (charts, models, written communication) to augment speech	• Try to give important information when the person is tired or stressed
• Don't change topics quickly	
• Ensure hearing aids, if used, are working properly (batteries usually need to be replaced every 1 to 2 weeks depending on use)	

to do it. So that perhaps he can see and then understand what I mean. Do not nag, they get tired. I want him to understand what I am going to do, with the face flannel for example, before I do it, I do not want to bully him, ride roughshod over him, I am afraid that he can not understand what my intentions are…I do not buzz around, instead for example, I just stretch his arm a bit so that he realizes himself what he should do, sometimes it can take ages before you get a response from the patient, he needs a lot of time (p. 112).[17]

Include social communication in your interactions and don't limit communication to just illness concerns.[24] Helpful communication strategies should be shared with all staff members who are caring for the person. Consistent caregivers who come to know the person and his or her needs will also facilitate better communication.

Dysarthria is a speech disorder that may be associated with Parkinson disease and multiple sclerosis. Dysarthria is caused by weakness or lack of coordination of the muscles used for speech. Dysarthric speech may be soft, slurred, jerky, breathy, and lacking in expression, making it very difficult to understand especially in noisy areas. Dysarthria does not affect a person's intelligence or understanding, so assume that you will communicate at an adult level. It is important to communicate in quiet areas and allow more time for conversation. Assessments may need to be divided into several sessions to prevent fatigue. Ask the person what you can do to improve communication. Finishing sentences may be welcomed. Offer the client the choice to write rather than speak. If you cannot understand his or her speech, be honest and tell the person, but keep trying. Seek validation of what you think you heard the person say. You can repeat the part of the message you didn't understand so the speaker does not have to repeat the whole message. Work with the speech language pathologist to assist in improving communication. Encouraging facial exercises such as pursing the lips, blowing, throwing kisses, and facial massage may be helpful strategies to enhance speech ability in a person with dysarthria. Other strategies are listed in Table 8-3. [25]

Table 8-3   Strategies for Clients Who Have Dysarthria

- Ask, "Do you need more time?"
- Ask permission to guess words.
- Encourage the client to use deep breathing to relax.
- Use humor to promote relaxation.
- Check your communication: "Am I making this clear?"
- Change topics slowly.
- Let the client know you are about to change topics.

■ CONCLUSIONS

Older adults are at risk for conditions that cause speech and language disorders. Age-related changes in the senses also affect communication. All senses gradually decline as people age. These normal changes of aging do not occur abruptly, and most people adapt fairly well. However, significant hearing, vision, speech, and language losses have the potential to affect the person's ability to understand and comprehend the world around them and can severely affect communication. The role of the nurse is to augment and maximize the elder's remaining abilities and to help design the environment to promote meaningful interaction.

To communicate effectively with all older clients, the nurse must work toward mutuality. Mutuality is a characteristic of therapeutic relationships in which there is respect, intimacy, and a sense of connection between nurse and client.[26] When there is mutuality in a relationship, there is shared responsibility between the client and nurse for the client's care. Communication reflects "understanding and intimacy," "joint ownership and mutual satisfaction," "give and take, exchange of ideas, respect for all possibilities, creativity, comfort, humor, and humanness" (p. 6).[26] Entering the lives of the elders you care for and sharing their wisdom can be enriching for both the nurse and the elder. Older people have much to share with those of us who will also be going on that journey.

REFERENCES

1. Campbell, S. (2007). Hear your soul speak to you. *Geriatric Nursing, 28*(1), 56.

2. Ebersole, P., Hess, P., Touhy, T., & Jett, K. (2005). *Gerontological nursing and healthy aging.* St. Louis, MO: Elsevier.

3. Rowe, J.W., & Kahn, R.L. (1998). *Successful aging.* New York: Pantheon Books.

4. Kiely, D.K., Simon, M.A., Jones, R.N., & Morris, J.N. (2000). The protective effect of social engagement on mortality in long-term care. *Journal of the American Geriatrics Society, 48,* 1367–1372.

5. Edwards, H., & Chapman, H. (2004). Contemplating, caring, coping, conversing: A model for promoting mental wellness in later life. *Journal of Gerontological Nursing, 30*(4), 16–21.

6. Miller, L. (2002). Effective communication with older people. *Nursing Standard, 17*(9), 45–50, 55.

7. Touhy, D. (2003). Student nurse-older person communication. *Nurse Education Today, 23*(1), 19–26.

8. Barker, V., Giles, H., & Harwood, J. (2004). Inter- and intragroup perspectives on intergenerational communication. In J.F. Nussbaum & J. Coupland (Eds.). *Handbook of communication and aging research* (2nd ed.). Mahwah, NJ: Lawrence Erlbaum Publishers.

9. Williams, K., Kemper, S., & Hummert, M.L. (2003). Improving nursing home communication: An intervention to reduce elderspeak. *The Gerontologist, 43*(2), 242–247.

10. Williams, K., Kemper, S., & Hummert, M.L. (2004). Enhancing communication with older adults: Overcoming elderspeak. *Journal of Gerontological Nursing, 30*(10), 17–25.

11. Kemper, S., & Harden, T. (1999). Experimentally disentangling what's beneficial about elderspeak from what's not. *Psychology and Aging, 14,* 656–670.

12. Van Etten, D. (2006). Psychotherapy with older adults: Benefits and barriers. *Journal of Psychosocial Nursing and Mental Health Services, 44*(11), 28–33.

13. Touhy, T. (2001). Touching the spirit of elders in nursing homes: Ordinary yet extraordinary care. *International Journal for Human Caring, 6*(1), 12–17.

14. Buckwalter, K.C., Gerdner, L.A., et al. (1995). Shining through: The humor and individuality of persons with Alzheimer's disease. *Journal of Gerontological Nursing, 21*(3), 11–16.

15. Murphy, J., Tester, S., Hubbard, G., & Downs, M. (2005). Enabling frail older people with communication difficulties to express views: The use of Talking Mats as an intervention tool. *Health and Social Care in the Community, 13*(2), 95–107.

16. National Institute on Aging. Chapter 2: Listening to older people. Retrieved February 20, 2007 from www.nia.nih.gov

17. Sundin, K., & Jansson, L. (2003). Understanding and being understood as a creative phenomenon in care of patients with stroke and aphasia. *Journal of Clinical Nursing, 12,* 107–116.

18. Boykin, A., Parker, M., & Touhy, T. (1998). Discovering the beauty of older adults: Opening doors. *Journal of Clinical Psychology, 4*(3), 205–210.

19. Sandelowski, M. (1994). We are the stories we tell. *Journal of Holistic Nursing, 12*(1), 23–33.

20. Coles, R. (1989). *The call of stories.* Boston: Houghton Mifflin Co.

21. Wallhegen, M., Pettengill, E., & Whiteside, M. (2006). Sensory impairment in older adults: Part 1 Hearing loss. *American Journal of Nursing, 106*(10), 40–48.

22. Crews, J.E., & Campbell, V.A. (2004). Vision impairment and hearing loss among community-dwelling older Americans: Implications for health and functioning. *American Journal of Public Health, 94*(5), 823–829.

23. Demers, K. (2001). Hearing screening. *Journal of Gerontological Nursing, 27*(11), 8–9.

24. Davidson, B., Worrall, L., & Hickson, L. (2006). Social communication in older age: Lessons from people with aphasia. *Topics in Stroke Rehabilitation, 13*(1), 1–13.

25. Nordehn, G., Meredith, A., & Bye, L. (2006). A preliminary investigation of barriers to achieving patient-centered communication with patients who have stroke-related communication disorders. *Topics in Stroke Rehabilitation, 13*(1), 68–77.

26. Henson, R.H. (1997). Analysis of the concept of mutuality. *Journal of Nursing Scholarship, 29*(1), 77–81.

EXERCISES

1. Self-Assessment

Working with aging adults can be both challenging and rewarding. Use these exercises to help you develop self-understanding about caring for older clients.

A. List 10 words that come to mind when you picture someone who is "old."

1.	6.
2.	7.
3.	8.
4.	9.
5.	10.

Are these words mostly positive or negative? As a result of this exercise, what have you learned about your beliefs about aging?

B. What do you think it means to be "healthy" in old age?

C. Feeling empathy for someone who is in late life can be difficult when our experiences seem so different. It may help to do the following exercise. Picture yourself at age 85.

What do you look like?

Where are you living?

With whom do you enjoy spending time?

What do you enjoy doing?

What is most important to you?

What are your greatest joys?

What brings you sadness?

What do you see as your major health problem?

Discussion

Write a brief summary of what you think it might be like to be old. If you were old, what would you like your nurse to do or say?

2. Responding to Situations

Below are situations in which you might find yourself as you interact with older adults in the clinical setting. These situations are posed to help you better understand the process of therapeutic interaction.

A. Your client, Mr. Snow, is 80 years old and was admitted to the hospital from home. His vision is adequate, but he has severe hearing impairment. When you visit him in his room to conduct your initial assessment, you note that he screams whenever you touch him.

What do you think Mr. Snow feels in this situation?

What might you feel in this situation?

What could you say or do to reduce Mr. Snow's anxiety and assess his pain?

B. Mrs. Alvarez, age 92, comes to an ambulatory center for diagnostic tests. She lives with her family. When you greet her, she does not respond. Her daughter tells you that she had a stroke one year ago and has difficulty speaking.

What would you do to communicate with Mrs. Alvarez?

What would be a good psychosocial outcome in this situation?

Discussion

In your self-assessment notebook, summarize what you have learned in doing this exercise. What kinds of feelings do you experience in caring for older people? How do you handle those feelings? What would you like to change about the way you approach older adult clients?

9

Communicating with Cognitively Impaired Persons

Christine L. Williams, DNSc, APRN, BC and Ruth M. Tappen, EdD, RN, FAAN

OBJECTIVES

1. To describe nurse and client responses to communication challenges related to cognitive impairment

2. To differentiate delirium, dementia, and intellectual/developmental disabilities

3. To delineate therapeutic communication strategies for clients with cognitive impairment

4. To compare and contrast task-focused and emotion-focused communication

5. To adjust communication approaches to the severity of the client's cognitive impairment

■ INTRODUCTION

Cognitive impairment may occur at any age and may be encountered in the home, clinic, or hospital.[1] Some types of impairment can be reversed, others cannot. In either case, cognitive impairment presents a communication challenge to the nurse.

One type of cognitive impairment is *dementia,* which is caused by degenerative brain disease, such as Alzheimer's disease (AD), and is usually not reversible.[2] Dementia is most common in older adults. *Intellectual and developmental disabilities* (I/DD) occur before birth or during childhood. They can be treated but usually are not reversible. Although considered a problem of childhood, as treatment of I/DD improves, nurses encounter many more adults with I/DD. *Delirium* is an acute, potentially reversible event that may occur at any age, although older

adults are most vulnerable. An estimated 20% of adults aged 65 and older who are hospitalized develop delirium.[3]

Because the communication strategies nurses implement with clients exhibiting these different types of cognitive impairment vary somewhat, they will be discussed separately.

■ DEMENTIA

Dementia is a gradual loss of cognitive ability that usually occurs during old age. Half of all older adults over the age of 85 have dementia.[2] It is never a normal or expected part of aging. Dementia occurs with brain pathology and must be evaluated to rule out other causes and determine if the dementia is reversible (e.g., vitamin B_{12} deficiency or thyroid disease). The most common form of dementia, Alzheimer's disease, is irreversible, but medications may slow the progression of the illness. Other causes of dementia include chronic alcoholism, stroke, and HIV.[3]

An individual with dementia gradually loses an array of cognitive abilities, such as memory, calculation, judgment, or orientation. Aphasia, or deteriorating language, is another common cognition-related loss. Anomia (word-finding difficulty) is one of the first signs. This is followed by difficulty verbally expressing thoughts and emotions, as well as difficulty in understanding verbal messages.[4] Cognitive losses gradually increase over a period of months or years. Although the individual remains alert, he or she eventually loses the ability to comprehend verbal communications. The result is a slower response to a question or command and frequent miscommunication.

■ NURSE AND CLIENT RESPONSES
TO COGNITIVE IMPAIRMENT

People with dementia were once cognitively intact. Clients' emotional responses to their cognitive loss will influence their overall mental health and ongoing relationships. As clients develop dementia, different cognitive abilities decline at different rates. They retain many cognitive abilities while other cognitive skills deteriorate. People who are painfully aware of their limitations may be reluctant to try to communicate. They may feel ashamed and withdraw from relationships or activities.[5]

Frustration, anger, and anxiety are common human responses for any individual who loses the ability to communicate verbally. When losses are gradual and relentless, such as in dementia, decreased self-esteem and depression are common and further interfere with the ability to communicate. With little hope for improvement and frequent awkward misunderstandings, it is not surprising that clients would wish to avoid communicat-

> ### Case example
>
> Mrs. Trescott, age 86, has lived a full and active life. She held positions of responsibility and enjoyed leadership status in her community. She has fond memories of winning her golf club championship several years in a row. Presently, she lives in a long-term care facility and has Alzheimer's disease. Although she is unable to live independently, she speaks about the indignities of living in a sheltered environment. She is embarrassed about attending group exercise classes because the routines are well below her ability level. At the same time, she can be loud and disruptive in social activities and must be closely supervised because she wants to leave the facility to go shopping on her own.

ing. Caregivers are also subject to frustration and anxiety when their attempts to communicate with the person who has cognitive limitations are unsuccessful. Mutual

Table 9-1   Guidelines for Communication with Cognitively Impaired Persons

Strategy	Explanation
Simplify your message Use common words and short sentences. Ask one question at a time.	Aphasia limits the person's ability to understand complex verbal messages.
Accept the client's message	People with dementia may confuse the date or use one word and mean another. By avoiding correcting mistakes, the nurse demonstrates supportiveness.
Allow extra time If there is no response, try repeating the message or use different words and gestures.	Cognitive impairment slows comprehension; wait for a response.
Break tasks down into simple steps Give instructions one step at a time.	Cognitive impairment interferes with remembering multiple steps.
Avoid the use of pronouns Repeat names so that your message is clear.	Cognitive impairment interferes with remembering the word or name to which the pronoun refers.
Use a calming approach	Conversation can be stressful. A soothing tone and an unhurried approach may prevent the client from feeling overwhelmed.
Take a break, try again later If you or the client becomes frustrated, try another approach at a later time.	Miscommunication can be trying for both the nurse and the person with dementia. Maintaining a warm and supportive relationship is of utmost importance.

avoidance and withdrawal can be the result.[6,7] Many strategies are available for nurses to use to increase their chances of successful communication with these clients (see Table 9-1).

As you develop knowledge and skill you will be more likely to approach cognitively impaired clients with confidence rather than unease. Approaches to communication must be adapted not only to the person's ability to understand and respond but to the purpose of the interaction. What is appropriate for assessment may be a barrier to conversation that is designed to facilitate expression of concerns and feelings.

■ BALANCING THE NEED TO KNOW WITH THE CLIENT'S NEED FOR DIGNITY

During the nurse's evaluation of the client's cognitive and communication abilities, the client's deficits are exposed. This exposure is frequently stressful and embarrassing to the client. It is important for the nurse to be especially supportive and to convey respect for the worth and dignity of the person. Prepare clients in advance for questions that may be difficult to answer. Let clients know that it is okay if they do not know the answer. Some people with dementia wonder aloud about the cause of their cognitive impairment and are self-critical. They may comment that they have become "stupid," "crazy," or they are "losing their mind." You can assure them that their memory problems do not have any relationship to such negative self-evaluations.

To provide safe and effective care, it is often necessary for the nurse to conduct an assessment of the client's cognitive ability. The Mini Mental State Examination (MMSE) is one test used to evaluate cognitive functioning in several areas including orientation, registration, attention and calculation, recall and language.[8] The MMSE is used in assessing clients with cognitive impairment as well as those who are at risk for dementia, such as older adults or those with HIV and chronic substance abuse. The test can be introduced to the individual as a routine series of questions—some of which may be easy and others difficult to answer. A person with dementia will be unable to answer some questions and will commonly react with discomfort and dismay. Therefore, the test-taking situation is less threatening for the client when the nurse has established a trusting relationship and time is allowed to establish rapport before the test begins.

Clients should be advised to do their best in answering assessment questions and should be assured that not knowing an answer does not necessarily mean that something is wrong. Because testing can be uncomfortable for people with cognitive impairment, such questions should be reserved for special purposes, including evaluation of clinical progress and research. Quizzing clients and thus exposing their deficits whenever care is given is not helpful because it can harm self-esteem. Quizzing is quite different from a therapeutic strategy designed to stimulate cognitive activity. If the goal of the interaction is maintaining or regaining cognitive function, it is more helpful to involve clients in conversation about topics they choose or in activities they enjoy.

■ ENGAGING THE CLIENT IN COMMUNICATION

The goals of communication for people with cognitive impairment include understanding the client's needs, sharing experiences, and engaging the client in his or her own care. Table 9-1 presents some general guidelines that will facilitate successful communication with clients who have cognitive impairment.

Reality orientation is a strategy that involves providing information to people with cognitive impairment to help them maintain contact with reality.[9] For example, the nurse uses reality orientation in the following statement: "Mr. Jeffrey, my name is Beverly Tomez and I am your nurse. Today is Wednesday, January 23rd, and you are in the hospital." This statement is intended to reduce anxiety by reinforcing orientation to time and place. Although this strategy is not harmful when used occasionally, it has limited usefulness for interacting with a person who has dementia.[9] Many people with dementia become embarrassed or frustrated when they realize that they have forgotten the date or where they are. Further, they are likely to forget the information in a few minutes; reminding them over and over again is not helpful. Displaying a clock and calendar where they can be easily seen is more useful (and less threatening) because the information is available when the person needs it.

Facilitating Trust

Establishing trust with a person who has dementia is a challenging but not impossible task. When a trusting relationship is established, the goals of care are much easier to achieve. The person with dementia will remember that you are trustworthy, although he or she may not remember all of the details of the experience that led to the feeling of trust.

Case example

You are a nurse in a long-term care facility and a resident has an appointment with a specialist in a location off the unit. The nursing assistant is trying to persuade the resident to accompany her to the appointment, and the resident is anxious and reluctant to get onto the elevator. Hoping to gain the resident's cooperation, the nursing assistant tells the resident that her son is waiting and she must get into the elevator if she wants to see him. What would you do?

The short-term effect of the dishonesty in the case example is that the resident may get into the elevator. Later, the person with dementia may become disruptive and uncooperative and will be unlikely to trust what the nursing assistant tells her. A better approach would be to encourage a trusted family member or consistent caregiver to be present at the time of the appointment, to allow extra time to accompany the resident, and to ensure that the caregiver uses a calming approach. If the resident becomes agitated upon leaving the unit, this is an issue that can be discussed with the family and interdisciplinary team. It may be possible for a small dose of an as-needed medication for anxiety to be given in advance of the appointment or perhaps the care provider can come to the unit for a meeting.

Avoid talking about the person with cognitive impairment in his or her presence. Address the client directly instead of speaking to a nearby family member or coworker. Use the client's formal name and ask what he or she would like to be called. Avoid endearments such as "Dear" or "Mamma," which imply a social relationship rather than a professional one. Remember, clients with dementia are adults, although some of their behavior may seem childlike.

Task-Focused Communication

When nurses request specific information from clients, such as, "Are you in pain?" or give directions, such as, "Take this medicine," they are using task-focused communication. The following approaches are guidelines for this type of interaction.

Because the individual may have difficulty understanding complex messages, keep your messages simple and direct. Present one idea at a time. Ask for what you want rather than what you do not want. For example, it is easier for people with dementia to understand a statement such as, "Hold the glass with both hands" than it is to understand and follow a negatively worded command such as, "Careful, don't spill your drink!"

Complex questions are also unlikely to produce a useful response. Asking two questions at once is confusing even to the person without cognitive impairment. Asking "why" requires analysis of reasons for behavior and sounds like a challenge or confrontation. For example, "Why did you put your coat on? It's hot outside!" This question is unlikely to produce a positive response. Instead, it would be better to preserve the person's sense of dignity with a supportive response. "Let me help you put your coat away. It is very hot out today. I don't think you will need it."

Do not overburden people with cognitive impairment with unnecessary information. In orienting them to a new living environment, for example, it may be more appropriate to include essential information about their immediate surroundings at first (such as where the bathroom is and how they can call for help) rather than an orientation to the entire unit. Allow for slower processing of information and give additional time for questions.

To gain your clients' cooperation, avoid increasing their anxiety. A statement such as, "If you can't stay in bed, I will have to put the side rails up!" is not likely to gain cooperation. Clients may not remember the details of such a threat a few minutes later, but they will feel less secure in their new surroundings. When the nurse remembers to plan care to accommodate people with cognitive deficits, less frustration will occur.

By giving simple choices and allowing some flexibility, the nurse empowers clients to participate in their care. For example, the nurse asks, "Would you like to wash your face?" (while handing the washcloth to the client), thereby encouraging the person to choose to participate rather than become the passive recipient of care. Do not pretend to provide a choice, however, if you are not able to accept a "no" response.

Arguing with someone who is cognitively impaired is unlikely to gain cooperation and will only escalate frustration and agitation. For example, Mrs. Silva shouts at the nursing assistant, "You stole my teeth!" Rather than defending herself and arguing that Mrs. Silva misplaced her own dentures, the nursing assistant wisely responds, "Let me help you find your dentures, Mrs. Silva."

Emotion-Focused Communication

Contrary to popular belief, clients with dementia can form therapeutic relationships with their nurses. Despite memory deficits, these clients have the same emotional needs as any other person including the need for relationships with others. In a study of nursing home residents with advanced dementia, nurses visited three times weekly over a period of 16 weeks.[5] During that time, residents remembered that they had a relationship with the nurses and frequently brought up what was discussed at previous sessions, although they may not have remembered the nurses' names. They also chose to discuss their emotions and concerns. Some of the topics included death, loneliness, isolation, and relationships with family members. It was not unusual for residents to discuss their feelings about the nurse (e.g., "I missed you!").

Care providers frequently assume that because cognitively impaired people have difficulty finding the words to express ideas, they have lost their individuality, their humanity, and, in some cases, their entire "self." This sense of who they are, in fact, persists over the course of the dementing illness.[7] Recognition of the person as a person is necessary to maintain quality of life.

Most communication is nonverbal; therefore nurses can understand much about a person by being observant. Feelings are conveyed with facial expressions, posture, tone of voice, and gestures. It is not necessary for clients to tell us in words that they are frightened or angry. Anxiety can be communicated with overall body tension or facial expressions such as worry lines, wide eyes, or eyes that seem to scan the environment for a threat. Anger may be portrayed by banging the hand on an object, yelling, or a tightly held fist. Slumped posture or the chin propped up with a hand may indicate dis-

couragement or depression. Many people with dementia who have limited speech become agitated and restless when they experience strong emotions. When agitation occurs, assume that the person is distressed and begin searching for the cause. Look for situational cues. What happened just before the person became agitated? Ask for validation of what you perceive (e.g., "You seem frightened.").

If the client has limited speech, assume that he or she hears and understands at least some of what is being communicated. Respect for the dignity of the person is conveyed in many subtle ways. If you relax and sit down before beginning a conversation, you convey "I have time for you." It may only be a few minutes, but you can give the individual your full attention for whatever time you have. The strategies listed in Table 9-2 can be used to guide the nurse in emotion-focused conversations with clients who are cognitively impaired.[6]

It is especially important to provide the healing presence of a nurse during important life changes and times of crisis. We can assume that people with dementia will have emotional responses to major events in their lives just as any other person would. If a long-time resident of an assisted living facility has to be moved to the nursing home due to increasing frailty, the nurse can assume that the resident will experience anxiety and loss and will be at risk for agitation and depression. In anticipation, the nurse needs to arrange opportunities for support. Spending time with the person who has dementia will provide the opportunity to observe and listen for the emotions expressed with or without words. Although the words in

Table 9-2   Guidelines for Emotion-Focused Communication

Strategy	Explanation
Making time	Sitting with the client, making eye contact, and using touch provides the atmosphere for emotion-focused conversation.
Being receptive	Acknowledging concerns and emotions encourages expression.
Broad openings	Beginning with general questions and statements encourages clients to choose what to talk about.
Speaking as equals	Relating to clients as people with something to offer in the relationship facilitates trust.
Establishing commonalities	Sharing experiences can be a way of developing and deepening the relationship between nurse and client.
Maintaining the conversation	Following up on important concerns and emotions facilitates the flow of conversation.

a conversation may be difficult to follow, emotions can be understood nonverbally, as discussed.

Allowing and even encouraging expression of negative emotions such as anger and grief can be therapeutic. People with dementia need to know that someone hears their distress and will be with them and respond with empathy. Too often, unpleasant emotions are dismissed by distracting cognitively impaired people with pleasant thoughts and activities. It is important to give them the opportunity to express their feelings and receive support. These periods of emotional expression can be balanced with pleasant activities as well. It is not therapeutic to deny painful feelings nor is it helpful to dwell on them to the exclusion of enjoying other activities.

Facilitating discussion of sensitive topics is important, but clients' limitations need to be considered as well. Clients who are cognitively intact remember painful events under discussion (such as the death of a loved one) and prior discussions of the event. People with cognitive impairment may react to discussion of painful events as if they are hearing about it for the first time. Being therapeutic involves adjusting your approach to this reality. The following case example illustrates this point.

Case example

An 89-year-old woman is wandering on the dementia unit and calling out for her husband, who died more than 10 years ago. She appears sad and anxious and is becoming agitated. One response might be to tell her that her husband is working and he will be home later that day. This explanation may even seem to calm her for the moment; however, a feeling of uncertainty and mistrust may result when the promised reunion does not occur.

Another approach to this situation is brutal honesty. Telling her that her husband passed away and that she now lives in a nursing home rather than with her husband may result in tearfulness and distress. With this response, the tears may be quieted with comforting, but the individual with memory loss may be calling out for her husband again a few minutes later.

Instead, it is possible to respond supportively without doing harm. If she misses her husband she may benefit by reminiscing about him. Ask her to tell you about her husband and about her life with him. This approach allows her to meet a need to remember her husband without cutting off discussion of this sensitive subject.

■ COMMUNICATION STRATEGIES FOR CLIENTS WITH DEMENTIA

In a study of communication strategies used by nurses, several strategies were identified as helpful in encouraging the expression of feelings in individuals with dementia.[6] Using *broad openings* is one strategy. A question as simple as, "How are you?" encourages discussion and allows the person to respond in whatever way he or she can to communicate concerns. It does not limit the client to a "yes" or "no" answer, as "Are you upset?" would.

Another successful strategy is referred to as *speaking as equals*. This means creating a climate of respect in which the interviewer views the client as someone to learn from and someone of equal value in the relationship. *Establishing commonalities* is another helpful strategy that means sharing perceptions or interests. The following case example illustrates sharing perceptions.

Case example

Mrs. Jackson, a 90-year-old resident of a dementia unit in a nursing home, has limited speech. The nurse spent a few minutes with Mrs. Jackson after another resident had become extremely agitated in the dining area and was led away. Mrs. Jackson remarked, "It's crazy in this place!" The nurse shares her perception that "it is very confusing here this morning."

Sharing of self involves the nurse offering his or her feelings or thoughts in the conversation with the person who has dementia. Positive feelings are expressed verbally or nonverbally with touch. When nurses share their feelings, they reinforce the idea that a valued relationship exists between two people.

Maintaining the conversation is a strategy that encompasses efforts to continue the interaction despite unclear verbalizations. Nurses listen for recurring themes in conversation and summarize what they hear to help people with dementia express concerns and emotions. By verbalizing themes and asking clients for validation, the nurse checks for accuracy of understanding. "You have been talking about all the things you miss about your home in Chicago. Are you feeling sad today?" Nurses use nonverbal and verbal encouragers (head nodding and "uh-huh") to assist clients to elaborate.

Nurses may be uncomfortable and may even avoid interaction when they do not understand people with dementia. Those with cognitive losses and accompanying communication deficits may avoid confronting their losses and withdraw as well. The nurse who is skilled in communicating can prevent clients' isolation and thus play an important role in enhancing quality of life for people with dementia.

ADJUSTING COMMUNICATION TO THE STAGE OF DEMENTIA

As clients move into the later stages of a dementing illness, communication strategies must be adapted to their declining language abilities. A decline in the number of words a client uses and in the relevance of responses are common. For some clients, verbalizations are long and repetitive and lack relevance to a topic. *Mutism* gradually occurs for others. This means speaking may become less and less frequent until verbal communication ceases. In the final stages of dementia, the individual seems unaware of his or her surroundings.[10]

As verbal abilities decline, the client must put forth greater and greater effort to communicate. Adjust the amount of time you expect the client to engage in conversation accordingly. Someone with minimal impairment may enjoy 30 minutes of conversation, while the individual with more severe impairment may only tolerate 15 minutes. Take your cues from the client. With regular opportunities to converse, most clients can increase the amount of time spent in conversation with a trusted caregiver.

During the later stages of dementia, it is still important to remember that the client may understand more than you realize. Continue to narrate what you do in a calming voice. Address the client by name and use gentle touch on an arm or shoulder to focus his or her attention. Use supportive facial expressions, such as smiling and eye contact. Use gestures to reinforce verbal messages. Assume the client can understand, and ask for his or her cooperation as you provide care. Many caregivers can relate experiences in which people with advanced dementia surprised them with an action or statement that indicated much more awareness than expected. Knowing that you have communicated successfully with someone who is difficult to reach is a very rewarding experience.[11]

DELIRIUM

Delirium is an acute decline in attention and cognitive function[3] accompanied by disturbance of consciousness, visual hallucinations, and communication difficulties. It occurs over a short period of time (hours or days) and is considered to be a medical emergency. The person's level of consciousness may change from alert to lethargic. A few hours later, he or she may be difficult to arouse or may be hyperalert. Inattentiveness and disorganized thinking are also common.[4,12]

Precipitating factors are medical illnesses or procedures resulting in hypoxia, toxic reactions to medication or other substances, anesthesia, dehydration, infection, and fever.[13] Older adults are especially vulnerable.[3] Rapid identification of the underlying problem is critical so that corrective action can be taken. To provide a feeling of safety for the client, the nurse should use a calming approach both verbally and nonverbally, thus limiting the anxiety that the client will inevitably experience in such a situation. Unhurried actions and a soothing tone of voice will contribute to the overall calming effect of the nurse's behavior. The guidelines for communication with cognitively impaired people identified in Table 9-1 are also appropriate to use with the person experiencing delirium.

A professional nurse should closely monitor such a client to prevent harm from agitated behavior and a rapidly changing condition. Speak to the client although you may not be sure you are heard and understood. Clients who have experienced delirium may tell you that they remember the nurse as a source of comfort and reassurance.

Disorganized thinking will limit the amount of information clients can comprehend. Remind clients of who you are and what they can expect to reduce anxiety caused by the unfamiliar situation. For example, "Mr. Brown, I am your nurse, Jeffrey Levine, you are in the hospital and I will be taking care of you today." As a client's condition changes, be prepared to alter your verbal approach. Use moments of increased alertness as opportunities to interact and reinforce orienting information.

Explain what you are doing, but use simple terms and repeat your message often. Encourage family members to sit with the client and provide touch and a calming presence. It is much better to use close observation by a person to maintain safety than it is to use restraints.[14] Help the client to explore tubes and lines with you as you guide his or her hands and briefly explain what he or she is touching. Move tubes and lines away from the client's field of vision to reduce the chance that he or she will pull at them during periods of clouded consciousness.

The methods described in this chapter for emotion-focused communication with people who have dementia are of limited use for people with delirium. The delirious client needs to trust that he or she is safe and is being cared for while every effort is made to identify and reverse the underlying problem that is causing the delirium. Consistent caregivers, gentle touch, patience, and a soothing tone of voice contribute to a feeling of security.

■ INTELLECTUAL AND DEVELOPMENTAL DISABILITIES

Infants, children, and adults with intellectual and developmental disabilities (I/DD) often have difficulty making themselves understood and understanding others. Their communication problems may be due to their intellectual limitations, to hearing or visual deficits, difficulty speaking (dysarthria), or even to movement disorders that limit their nonverbal responses. The range of cognitive impairment is very wide, from mildly to profoundly impaired.

Each individual, whether child or adult, has his or her own unique combination of strengths and limitations.[14] An assessment of these strengths and limitations should guide the nurse's choice of communication strategies.

Mental retardation is a disability occurring before age 18 that is characterized by significant limitations in intellectual functioning and in adaptive behaviors.[15] It is very important to help those who are severely intellectually disabled to express themselves and make their needs known. With the very young, whose communication skills are still developing, you can imitate the sounds they make and copy their expressions to establish a basis for two-way communication. Later on, pictures, objects, pointer boards (boards with pictures of basic needs such as a glass of water, food, or toilet, or numbers and the alphabet for those with higher intellectual skills but limited speech), and electronic devices may be used to supplement or encourage verbal communication. They may be used to communicate a need such as thirst or help getting to the toilet, to practice naming, or as a basis for conversation.

To help the severely intellectually disabled child or adult understand what is being said, you can use many

---

Case example

Terry became very anxious, trying to climb over the tray holding him in his chair, crying out and rocking back and forth. The nursing aide brought him his pointer board. He looked at it and started banging hard on the picture of the toilet. The aide quickly helped him into the bathroom and he visibly relaxed as he emptied a very full bladder.

---

of the strategies listed in Table 9-1. Try to simplify what you are saying. Emphasize the most important words and avoid verbal clutter. If you do not know the client's level of comprehensive ability, begin with a full but basic sentence such as, "Tanya, do you want some milk?" Allow lots of time for a response (take a deep breath and slowly exhale), repeat your question, and allow more time for a response. Repeat a third time if needed. If your sentence is too complex, simplify it more, reducing it to only the words needed to convey the purpose of your question: "Want milk?" If there still is no response, bring a glass of milk to Tanya and offer it to her both verbally and nonverbally.

If the client can engage in more complex conversation, begin with the "here and now" and concrete rather than abstract topics[16] such as people in the same room, the rain you can see out the window, a photo album, or a favorite article in the room. Focus on the client's interests, whether it's movies, sports, dolls, animals, etc. Gently challenge the client's ability to respond, making the conversation more complex or abstract a little at a time, but gradually enough to avoid failure and frustration. Progress will be made by inches and some regression can be expected on "bad" days.

One of the ways in which we hold someone's attention during a conversation is through the use of eye contact. The use of eye contact may not develop spontaneously in some children with autism and other I/DDs. Instead, some may watch the person's mouth or hands as they speak. By gently placing a finger under the child's chin, you can direct his or her attention upward.

Case example

In a small class of 5-year-olds with I/DDs, Ms. Bea often used touch to gain a child's attention, especially a touch under the chin. Robert desperately wanted to get Ms. Bea to notice a big bug crawling under the table but couldn't tell her, so he walked around the table to where she was seated, put his finger under her chin, and said "Ms. Bea!"

■ ESTABLISHING ROUTINES AND CUEING

Clear, simple routines for accomplishing basic everyday tasks provide consistency, security, manageability, and increased independence for a child or adult with I/DD. Begin by setting regular times for washing, toileting, eating, and dressing. Encourage your client to learn the basic steps for each of these tasks. Cueing is another tool that can be employed to aid clients with I/DD. A cue is a memory aid (hint) that can be verbal or nonverbal. An example of a verbal cue is sounding out the first syllable of a word to help the client remember the word. A nonverbal cue could be placing a sign with a picture of a toilet and the word "toilet" on the bathroom door to remind memory-impaired clients of where the toilet is.

The degree of intellectual and physical ability will affect how much cueing and support will be needed and how long it will take to accomplish all of this. Provide enough assistance to avoid frustration and the almost inevitable loss of control that follows. Provide ample visual cues: lay out clothes in the order they're to be put on, or, even better, create a big picture chart to do the same. Label items with pictures or words, everything from the sock drawer to the cabinet where cereal is kept to assist in locating them independently.

Remember the difference in the purposes of task- and emotion-focused communication. Visual cues are task-focused communications in which getting something done is the primary goal. For these tasks, there is considerable value in creating routines based on visual cues and easily remembered sequences rather than a person-centered routine. If the routine is person-centered (only a relative or special staff member knows the client's routines), when that person is unavailable, your client becomes lost.

A hospitalization, relocation to a residential facility, or even a medical procedure interferes with these carefully established routines. This can be extremely distressing. Every effort should be made to incorporate as much of the established routines as possible under the circumstances. In residential settings, the use of visual cues can decrease residents' disorientation and improve their ability to find their rooms (by displaying personal items at the entrance to the resident's room), or pictorial reminders can be used to decrease episodes of incontinence by orienting the individual to the location of the bathroom.

■ ESTABLISHING CONTACT AND BUILDING TRUST

The nurse needs to establish a connection with both the family and child or young adult with I/DD. Begin with mutual respect; while the nurse has professional expertise, the parents have experience caring for their offspring. Thorough discussion with the parents of the child's routines, means of communication, particular fears, and sources of comfort, is essential. The child or young adult knows what he or she wants and what he or she fears. His input, even if nonverbal, must also be respected.

Families may "test" the nurse for trustworthiness.[16] They need to know that the nurse recognizes the uniqueness and individuality of their child. They also need to know that the child's needs will be met, that a sobbing child will not be ignored, and that a meal will not be left to grow cold if they are not present because their child cannot call for help. Parents of children with I/DD are especially sensitive to any hint of blame or condescension. They will quickly recognize if they are just being placated. Most will be very anxious, upset that their child needs hospitalization, and stressed by this and other demands on their time and attention. Genuine listening, without impatience, without prejudgment, is the only way to earn their trust and to eventually develop a partnership with them to provide the best care for their child.

Down syndrome is the most common genetic cause of mental retardation. It is usually diagnosed at birth. Physical characteristics include a flattened face with upslanted eyes, epicanthal folds, a small mouth with protruding tongue, short neck, and small hands with short, incurved "pinky" fingers. Infants may not suck vigorously.[15] Children and adults with Down syndrome have low normal to profoundly impaired intellectual levels. They may also have low levels of muscle tone that results in relatively weak or muted responses to attempts to communicate nonverbally. This is especially disappointing for some parents, discouraging their attempts to communicate if they're not aware of this problem. It may also be hard to hold the child's attention and understand his or her speech. On the positive side, most individuals with Down syndrome do develop speech. In the interim, many benefit from learning how to use sign language and other nonverbal forms of communication.[17] A drawback of signing that the nurse should be aware of is that most people cannot interpret the signs, thus frustrating the signer if parents or caregivers do not help with interpretation.

Children and adults with autism spectrum disorders (ASD) present a different picture. ASDs are developmental disabilities characterized by substantial impairment in social interaction and communication and the presence of unusual ways of learning, paying attention, and reacting to various stimuli. It usually appears before 3 years of age. Intellectual capacity can range from severely challenged to gifted.[18] A recent study by the Centers for Disease Control and Prevention found that 1 in

150 eight-year-old children across the United States have an ASD.[19] Although children with autism may speak relatively early, often it is simple repeating or "parroting" of what they hear (called echolalia) rather than spontaneous communication. Both children and adults with autism seem to take pleasure in repetitive, solitary activities, especially those that provide some type of sensory stimulation (humming, rocking, and spinning). They also have limited ability to empathize with others, which can have a profound effect on their social relationships. The result is that they live in a world seen as a "myriad of detail." Cognitive skill in generalizing, seeing patterns, and being able to categorize objects or ideas can be very limited. Szatmari[20] suggests that caregivers try to see the world through the autistic person's eyes but also to help him or her enter our world through gentle challenges, asking for more than the client has already done, and helping them adapt to our social world. He offers the following example.

> Stephen has been interested in wasps for several years. He talks about them all the time, with his teachers, his parents and grandparents, even with complete strangers. He catches wasps in a bottle and then releases them in his bedroom and enjoys watching them fly around the room. . . . At first Stephen's parents were completely bewildered by his interest in wasps and not a little upset. . . . But now they . . . have acquired a detailed knowledge of the wasp's habits and life span. The four of us sit and talk about wasps as if we are all entomologists attending some esoteric conference about the mating habits of yellow jackets. Stephen's disability has transformed us all (p. 3–4).

Stephen's story is one of adaptability on the part of his parents and therapist. To connect with him, they have entered his world. In doing so, they also provided him with an opportunity to socialize in a way that is comfortable, even pleasurable, for him.

■ CONCLUSION

Communicating with clients who are cognitively impaired is challenging. Cognitively impaired clients may resist care because they are frightened or depressed. It is important to develop trust and to avoid the use of force in providing care. The use of mechanical restraints has been shown to cause significant harm emotionally and physically, and the consequences may persist long after the episode has ended.[14] If combative behavior or resistance to care occurs, ask for help from the interdisciplinary team. A consult from a psychiatrist will be necessary to determine the appropriate medication for severe psychiatric symptoms and combativeness. Develop a consistent approach so that nurses on every shift will respond to these clients consistently.

■ ACKNOWLEDGMENT

The authors wish to thank Ms. Susan Purtic, Broward County School System, for sharing her perspectives on I/DD.

■ REFERENCES

1. Hendrix-Bedalow, P.M. (2000). Alzheimer's dementia: Coping with communication decline. *Journal of Gerontological Nursing, 26*(8), 20–24.

2. Small, G.W., Rabins, P.V., Barry, P.P., et al. (1997). Diagnosis and treatment of Alzheimer's disease and related disorders: Consensus statement of the American Association for Geriatric Psychiatry, the Alzheimer's Association, and the American Geriatrics Society. *Journal of the American Medical Association, 278*, 1363–1371.

3. Inouye, S.K., & Ferucci, L. (2006). Elucidating the pathophysiology of delirium and the interrelationship of delirium and dementia. *Journal of Gerontology: Medical Sciences, 61A*(12), 1277–1280.

4. American Psychiatric Association. (2000). *Diagnostic and statistical manual of mental disorders* (4th ed., text revision, DSM IV-TR). Washington, DC: Author.

5. Williams, C., & Tappen, R. (1999). Can we create a therapeutic relationship with nursing home residents in the later stages of Alzheimer's disease? *Journal of Psychosocial Nursing and Mental Health Services, 37*(3), 1–8.

6. Tappen, R., Williams-Burgess, C., Edelstein, J., Touhy, T., & Fishman, S. (1997). Communicating with individuals with Alzheimer's disease: Examination of recommended strategies. *Archives of Psychiatric Nursing, 11*(5), 249–256.

7. Tappen, R., Williams, C., Fishman, S., & Touhy, T. (1999). Persistence of self in advanced Alzheimer's disease. *Image: The Journal for Nursing Scholarship, 31*(2), 121–125.

8. Folstein, M.F., Folstein, S.E., & McHugh, P. (1975). "Mini-Mental State": A practical method for grading the cognitive state of patients for the clinician. *Journal of Psychiatric Research, 12,* 189–198.

9. Beck, C.K., & Shue, V.M. (1994). Interventions for treating disruptive behavior in demented elderly people. *Nursing Clinics of North America, 29*(1), 143–155.

10. Olga, V., & Emery, B. (2000). Language impairment in dementia of the Alzheimer's type: A hierarchical decline? *International Journal of Psychiatry in Medicine, 30*(2), 145–164.

11. Edberg, A.K., Nordmark, A., Sandgren, A., & Hallberg, I.R. (1995). Initiating and terminating verbal interaction between nurses and severely demented patients regarded as vocally disruptive. *Journal of Psychiatric and Mental Health Nursing, 2,* 159–167.

12. Henry, M. (2002). Descending into delirium. *American Journal of Nursing, 102*(3), 49–56.

13. Spar, J.E., & LaRue, A. (2002). *Concise guide to geriatric psychiatry* (3rd ed.). Washington, DC: American Psychiatric Association.

14. Rogers, P.D., & Bocchino, N.L. (1999). Restraint-free care: Is it possible? *American Journal of Nursing, 99*(10), 27–34.

15. Nehring, W. (2005). *Core curriculum for specializing in intellectual and developmental disability.* Sudbury, MA: Jones and Bartlett Publishers.

16. Warner, H.K. (2006). *Meeting the needs of children with disabilities: Families and professionals facing the challenge together.* New York: Routledge.

17. Launonen, K. (2003). Manual signing as a tool of communicative interaction and language: The development of children with Down syndrome and their parents. In S. VanTetzchner & Z. Grove, *Augmentative and alternative communication: Developmental issues* (pp. 83–122). London: Whurr Publishers.

18. Centers for Disease Control and Prevention. (2007a). Autism Information Center. Retrieved February 9, 2007 from http://www.cdc.gov/ncbddd/autism/overview.htm

19. Centers for Disease Control and Prevention. (2007b). *Prevalence of ASDs in multiple areas of the United States. Surveillance years 2000 and 2002. Morbidity and mortality weekly report surveillance summary.* Retrieved February 9, 2007 from www.cdc.gov/ncbddd/dd/addmprevalence.htm

20. Szatmari, P. (2004). *A mind apart: Understanding children with autism and Asperger syndrome.* New York: The Guilford Press.

EXERCISES

1. Self-Assessment

Working with cognitively impaired clients can be both challenging and rewarding. Use these exercises to help you develop self-understanding about caring for this population.

A. List 10 words that come to mind when you picture someone who is "senile."

1.   6.

2.   7.

3.   8.

4.   9.

5.   10.

As a result of this exercise, what have you learned about dementia and delirium that surprised you?

B. What do you think it means to be "confused" in old age?

C. Feeling empathy for someone who is confused can be difficult when she or he is hard to "manage." It may help to do the following exercise. Picture yourself at age 85. You have had minor surgery and you wake up from anesthesia confused. You scream for help but no one comes.

What might you feel in this situation?

What are you most afraid of?

What and who would you want to comfort you?

2. Responding to Situations

Below are situations in which you might find yourself as you interact with clients who have cognitive impairments in the clinical setting. These situations are posed to help you better understand the process of therapeutic interaction.

A. Your client, Mr. Schneider, is 90 years old and was admitted to the hospital from the nursing home with severe health problems including severe confusion. When you visit him in his room to conduct an initial assessment, you note that he screams whenever you touch him.

What do you think Mr. Schneider feels in this situation?

What could you say and do that might be helpful for Mr. Schneider?

B. Mrs. Jacobs, age 87, was admitted to the hospital for repair of a fractured hip. She fell at home where she lives with her family. You are the evening nurse assigned to her care. You notice that she seems confused, although this was not mentioned in the shift report. She is crying but does answer your questions about pain.

What might you be feeling in this situation?

What would be a good outcome in this situation?

Is there really anything that you can do that will help?

Discussion

In your self-assessment notebook, summarize what you have learned in doing this exercise. What kinds of feelings do you experience in caring for older people with cognitive impairments? How do you handle those feelings? What would you like to change about the way you approach elders with cognitive impairment?

10

Communicating with Critically Ill, Mechanically Ventilated Clients

Nancy E. Villanueva, PhD, ARNP, BC, CNRN

OBJECTIVES

1. To examine the barriers to communication that exist when caring for mechanically ventilated clients

2. To discuss the importance of communication from the client's perspective

3. To describe methods or techniques that may assist the nurse to communicate with mechanically ventilated patients

◼ INTRODUCTION

As discussed throughout this book, effective communication is essential to the relationship between the nurse and client. The ability to communicate is often taken for granted, and it is not appreciated until the nurse finds him- or herself in a situation in which the traditional means of communication are not possible. Nurses who practice in an intensive care unit provide care to clients who are unable to communicate verbally or nonverbally. For the client who is mechanically ventilated without cognitive impairment, the ability to speak is lost, but nonverbal communication remains possible. In contrast, the client who has a cognitive impairment (e.g., unconsciousness) and is mechanically ventilated has lost both verbal and nonverbal communication.

◼ VOICELESSNESS

Voicelessness has been identified as the inability to speak resulting from respiratory tract intubation and/or

mental status changes (permanent or transient).[1] Clients who have experienced voicelessness describe feelings of insecurity, frustration, anxiety, fear, anger, agony, and panic.[2-5] Asking a question or expressing a need is a challenge for the intubated client. In one study 29 clients were interviewed about their experience while intubated. Sixty-two percent of the clients reported high levels of frustration associated with their inability to communicate. Only 14% reported their experiences in communicating as not frustrating.[6] Trying to get the nurse to understand what the client is asking for can be an exhausting and frustrating experience. This sense of frustration can be seen in the following client's statement: "I can remember getting cross with everybody, getting cross with . . . my husband, my sister, my mum and dad because they couldn't understand what I was to say to them."[5] In another study, 13 of the 22 clients interviewed felt the registered nurse caring for them was able to understand their needs and wishes.[7]

Other frustrations arise from insufficient explanations and inadequate understanding of conversations with caregivers. Explanations related to the client's care and treatments are not clearly understood, and the client is unable to communicate the need for additional information and clarification. Also frustrating is the inability of the nurse to interpret the client's nonverbal cues, which result in misunderstanding of the client's request or continued attempts to communicate.[1,5,8] One nurse stated "I think it is one of the most frustrating things that can happen to a patient. The patient is lying there, completely helpless, trying to communicate desperately with you, and you have to say, 'No, I don't understand, sorry.'"[9]

■ BARRIERS TO COMMUNICATION WITH THE CRITICALLY ILL

The intensive care unit presents many barriers to effective nurse–client communication. Bassett[9] placed the various barriers in two categories: mechanical and psychological. Included in the mechanical category is the client's inability to speak or communicate. Factors that influence this category include the client's medical condition, the administration of sedating and neuromuscular blocking agents (NMBAs), presence of an artificial airway, and the noise generated by the various pieces of equipment and personnel in the intensive care unit.

Communication is an active process that requires energy. The client who is critically ill may not have the energy necessary to communicate or may only have a limited reserve that becomes depleted with repeated attempts to communicate. This is seen in a statement by a client: "He [nurse] tried very hard to communicate. He would watch my lips and mouth, because I couldn't use the [alphabet] board very well. I was so weak, and I forgot how to spell, just couldn't seem to get it all together, I was so groggy."[3]

The medications utilized also influence the ability to communicate. NMBAs are frequently employed in the care of the critically ill client. These agents paralyze the skeletal muscles and render the individuals unable to move or even open their eyes. For these clients, verbal and nonverbal communication is lost. The administration of sedating agents to mechanically ventilated clients also affects their ability to communicate by altering their mental status.[10]

■ FACTORS INFLUENCING NURSE–CLIENT COMMUNICATION

There are factors that may both limit and facilitate communication with intubated clients depending on the situation. Some of the factors identified by critical care nurses that limit their ability to communicate include:[1,3,8,10–12]

- The acuity of the client

- The individual nurse's assignment

- Inability to speak the client's language

- Difficulty reading the client's lips

- Inability of the client to write and/or read

- Continuity of client assignments

- Experience level of the nurse

- Presence of family and/or significant others

- Insufficient training in communication skills

Additional factors were identified when the client was comatose or unresponsive due to NMBAs. These factors included self-consciousness on the part of the nurse, lack of privacy, and the circumstances surrounding the injury. The nurses who were interviewed described feeling self-conscious talking to a client who was unable to talk back or use nonverbal methods. The majority of communication with clients consisted of informing them of upcoming procedures or activities. Rarely were nonprocedural topics discussed.[10]

The experience level of the nurse is a factor that can also inhibit communication. A grounded theory study by Villanueva[10] explored the experiences of critical care nurses caring for clients who were comatose due to a traumatic head injury or receiving NMBAs. As novices, the nurses described themselves as being task oriented, overwhelmed, and intimidated. Their focus was on managing the complex equipment and required nursing responsibilities. It was not until novices achieved a comfort level with the technical aspects of their role that they were able to focus on talking to clients. The client's acuity was also a factor in inhibiting communication even for experienced nurses. The higher the client's acuity, the greater the intensity required for monitoring physiological and neurological status, maintaining the complex equipment, and performing the numerous nursing responsibilities. As a result, the nurses talked less to their clients, and when they did talk, the conversation was limited to information about upcoming procedures or activities.

In a study by Patak,[6] practitioner interventions and attributes that promoted or inhibited communication were identified by previously mechanically ventilated patients. Attributes that were found to be helpful were being kind and patient, offering verbal reassurance and important information, and being present and available at the bedside. Characteristics and attributes that negatively impacted communication were providers who were described as mechanical, nonpersonal, inconsistent, inattentive, and "absent."

Additional factors that have been found to facilitate communication with the client include the client's ability to interact using nonverbal techniques and knowing about the client as a person. The presence of family and/or significant others allow the nurse to come to know the client as a person. Through interactions with the family, the nurse is able to learn about the client and his or her life. This information allows the nurse to provide individualized communication when talking to the client. An example of this can be seen in the following situation. The nurse knows from the family that the client is an avid sports fan, and when talking to the client, the nurse will include information related to recent sports events (e.g., Sunday football games and scores).[8,10,13] The presence of family can also assist in helping the nurse understand the client's nonverbal gestures and facial expressions, and they frequently are able to more easily interpret what the client is trying to communicate. Also, the family may be able to read the client's lips more clearly than the nurse.[8]

In two grounded theory studies, experienced intensive care nurses identified "maintaining continuity in client assignments" as a factor that promotes communication with clients. Having continuity in assignments allowed the nurses to come to know the client's nonverbal behaviors, facial expressions, and moods. Having this knowledge allowed them to be able to interpret what the client was trying to say more effectively and accurately.[10,14]

■ AUGMENTATIVE COMMUNICATION METHODS

A variety of communication tools can be utilized with the intubated client. The tools that are currently available require the client to be awake, alert, and have effective cognitive function. Other requirements are dependent on the tool selected.

Tools range from simple to complex devices. Tools that are frequently used include writing tablets, Magic Slates (Vic Enterprises, Tacoma, Washington), alphabet cards, alphabet boards, and picture boards. All of these tools require the client to have sufficient energy, writing or pointing ability, vision, and concentration to use the tool. Keep in mind that the intubated client has restricted head movement due to the endotracheal tube and ventilator tubing. This restriction may limit the use of some communication tools. The need for corrective lenses must also be addressed for the client to be able to see the tool being used.[3,12,13,15]

Another factor that must be taken into account when considering these tools is the client's ability to move an arm to point or ability to hold a pencil. Invasive monitoring lines, immobilization, or paralysis may restrict movement.[15]

In one study, a Magic Slate was used in an attempt to improve communication for clients with tracheostomies. Fifteen clients were asked to evaluate the effectiveness of the slate as a communication tool. Results showed that 73% of the clients felt that the tool was appropriate for their condition; 86% felt that it facilitated communication with the health care team; and the slate was accepted by 96% of the clients.[16]

An alphabet card and/or picture board can be used for clients who do not possess the ability to write or point. The picture board can also be used when the nurse does not speak the client's language. Alphabet cards are available commercially or may be written out by the nursing staff. The size is usually 8" × 12" and the letters are arranged in rows. To use the card, the nurse points to a line and asks the client if the word begins with a letter on that line. If the letter is not on that line, the nurse points to the next line and asks the same question. When the correct line is determined, the nurse points to each letter in the line. The client can indicate that the nurse has pointed to the correct letter by nodding his or her head or, if unable to move the head, by blinking his or her eyes. Spelling out a word using this technique is time consuming and can be frustrating for the client as well as the nurse. If the client has the ability to point to the letters, time and frustration can be reduced.[13]

Picture boards contain icons that depict a variety of basic needs to which the client points to express his or her needs to the nurse. Icons represent pain, hot and cold, thirst, and bedpan. Improvement in client–nurse communication was demonstrated in a study that utilized a picture board for intubated clients following cardiothoracic surgery.[13]

There are a variety of electronic voice output communication aids (VOCAs) that produce prerecorded, digitized voice messages (recorded speech) or synthesized speech (computer-generated voice). The devices may have a touch sensitive screen in which the client touches the icon that represents what he or she is trying to communicate. Touch-sensitive keyboards are also utilized. Examples of preprogrammed messages include "I am having pain," and "What time is it?" If possible, preoperative preparation allows the client to record messages using his or her own voice. In addition to standard messages, the client can add personalized ones. The devices can be mounted on an arm that is attached to the client's arm, or it can be hand held.[13,17]

The use of VOCAs by children was developed at the Children's Hospital in Boston for clients who remained intubated following surgery. Prior to surgery, the clients and family members selected and recorded items. These items were then stored as words or icons. If a preoperative visit was not possible, instruction was provided prior to the client receiving sedation. After the surgery is completed and the client is alert and able to use the device, the speech pathologist is contacted. The speech pathologist will make any modifications necessary for the device. Clients who participated in this model reported that they did not feel isolated, afraid, or exhausted while attempting to communicate because of communication problems.[17]

A pilot study involving the use of VOCA by 11 adult clients in a medical intensive care unit was conducted to describe the usage patterns, user perceptions, and characteristics of intubated clients who used VOCAs.[12] Results revealed that VOCA was not used as the dominant method of communication, and it was used more often by visitors than nurses. The device used was hand held, and most clients required some assistance (e.g., repositioning, cueing). Clients reported significantly less difficulty with communication after using the device. Families were positive about using the device and found the client easier to understand when the VOCA was utilized. Barriers to VOCA use were also identified. These included poor device repositioning (failure to replace or reposition the device after performing care), deterioration or fluctuation in the client's condition (motor and/or cognitive function), staff time constraints, staff lack of familiarity with the device, and device complexity (multilevel message screens).[12]

For clients with tracheotomies who meet the necessary criteria, a one-way Passy-Muir speaking valve is available. The one-way valve directs the exhaled air around the tracheotomy tube, through the vocal cords, and into the oral and nasal cavities, allowing the client to speak. A consultation with a speech pathologist is required for client evaluation to determine readiness for use of the tube. Absolute contraindications include foam-cuffed tracheotomy tubes, inflated tracheotomy cuffs, laryngectomy, sleep, or coma. Apraxia, oral motor weakness, or dysarthria are conditions that exclude the client as a candidate. Respiratory muscle strength, secretions, and oxygenation must also be taken into consideration. The length of time the valve is used increases as the client develops tolerance for the device. While the valve is in use, the nurse monitors the client's vital signs, oxygen saturation, work of breathing, and respiratory rate. The nurse collaborates with the respiratory therapist, who must adjust the ventilator settings to compensate for volume losses, F_iO_2, (Fraction of Inspired Oxygen) and positive end-expiratory pressure (PEEP). In addition to providing the ability to speak, the valve was found to improve swallowing skills, decrease secretions, and reestablish a sense of smell.[18,19]

A survey of 53 ventilator users was conducted to determine the nature of the communication challenges associated with ventilator use. The time associated with ventilator use ranged from 0.5 to 48.5 years. Communication strategies that were utilized included picture/word board, pen and pencil, lipreading, speaking valve, and VOCA. These individuals indicated that the most successful modes of communication involved the use of VOCAs or sign language/gestures.[20]

◼ IMPLICATIONS FOR NURSING PRACTICE

The importance of communication between nurses and mechanically ventilated clients has been well established along with the difficulties encountered when trying to communicate. Nurses need to recognize the impact that voicelessness has on clients. By putting him- or herself in the client's place, the nurse is able to experience voicelessness.

Nurses must also recognize that gestures, facial expressions, body language, and space all affect meaning. In addition, the tone of voice, pitch, and cadence influence the interpretation of a statement.[21,22] The opportunity to reposition a client for face-to-face communication may be limited by physiological status, monitoring devices, and intravenous tubing. Nevertheless, allowing the client to view the nurse during communication attempts will improve the chances of a successful interaction.

In a study in which nurses explored the client's experience of being mechanically ventilated, researchers identified five interventions that can improve the client's care. First each nurse must recognize the level of frustration the client feels when intubated. Second, clients should be routinely asked about their feelings and state of mind, permission should be obtained prior to commencing nursing procedures, and understanding should be verified with the use of yes/no questions. Third, nurses should inform clients about their surroundings and plan of care and establish a return time when leaving the bedside. Fourth, approach the client with a kind and patient manner, investigate their communication needs, and provide them with what is needed. Fifth, provide writing material and read the client's words as they write.[6]

Two strategies that may be utilized to determine if the nurse correctly understands what the client is attempting to communicate are: (1) look at the client's expression for evidence of relief or recognition, and (2) repeat back to the client what the nurse understands the client to be communicating. The client will indicate by a preestablished yes/no response if the message was correctly interpreted.[23]

When obtaining the client's history, it is important to determine if he or she wears eyeglasses (reading or distance) or has problems with hearing. Glasses may need to be modified to accommodate the client's condition. Take, for example, the client who has excessive head swelling or a head dressing. In both of these situations, the arms of the eyeglass frames will not fit. The arms can be removed and the glasses worn as spectacles. If the client has problems with hearing, is one ear better than the other? Or is a hearing aid used? If there is a hearing aid, it needs to be available for the client's use. The family should be asked to bring it from home. If the client is unable to wear the hearing aid, it may be helpful to consult the speech language pathologist to determine the availability of an auditory trainer/amplifier to assist the client.[17]

Nurses must recognize that family members or significant others may require support for facilitation of verbal communication with an intubated or sedated client. This need for support was identified in a study by Williams[8] and is expressed by a nurse's statement that "they sit at the end of the bed and are afraid to talk, and I say 'tell them about your family, what's going on, I'm sure they would like to know'" (p. 11).

Whenever possible, communication tools should be a standard part of the preoperative education for clients who will be mechanically ventilated after surgery. The client has the opportunity to practice using the selected tool prior to surgery. This provides a way for the client to communicate and decreases the feelings of insecurity, frustration, anxiety, fear, anger, agony, and panic that have been described by clients experiencing voicelessness.

In situations in which preoperative instruction is not possible, the nurse may select the communication tool best suited for the client. Nurses may consult and collaborate with speech language pathologists regarding the most appropriate tool for the client. The use of communication tools requires nurses to become knowledgeable and comfortable working with these devices.

◾ CONCLUSION

Communicating with an individual who is critically ill presents unique challenges for the nurse. Nurses must recognize the importance that communication represents for the client. The need to provide a way to achieve this communication should be given high priority. However, at times, the acuity of the client's psychological status requires the nurse's complete focus, and communication is limited to only the essential or technical aspects at that time. The voicelessness that accompanies mechanical ventilation is a common type of communication barrier requiring knowledge and skill to overcome. An experienced, competent nurse is better able to provide physical care while maintaining a focus on the client as a person. Advance planning when possible and augmentative communication devices can facilitate development and maintenance of a relationship with a mechanically ventilated client.

REFERENCES

1. Happ, M.B. (2000). Interpretation of nonvocal behavior and the meaning of voicelessness in critical care. *Social Science & Medicine*, 1247–1255.

2. Adamson, H., Murgo, M., Boyle, M., et al. (2004). Memories of intensive care and experiences of survivors of a critical illness: An interview study. *Intensive & Critical Care Nursing, 20*, 257–263.

3. Johnson, P. (2004). Reclaiming the everyday world: How long-term ventilated patients in critical care seek to gain aspects of power and control over their environment. *Intensive and Critical Care Nursing, 20*, 190–199.

4. Rotondi, A.J., Lakshmipathi, C., Sirio, C., et al. (2002). Patients' recollections of stressful experiences while receiving prolonged mechanical ventilation in an intensive care unit. *Critical Care Medicine, 30*(4), 746–752.

5. Todres, L., Fulbrook, P., & Albarran, J. (2000). On the receiving end: A hermeneutic-phenomenological analysis of a client's struggle to cope while going through intensive care. *Nursing in Critical Care, 5*(6), 277–287.

6. Patak, L., Gawlinski, G., Fung, N.I., et al. (2004). Patients' reports of health care practitioner interventions that are related to communication during mechanical ventilation. *Heart & Lung, 33*(5), 308–320.

7. Wojnicki-Johansson, G. (2001). Communication between nurse and client during ventilator treatment: Client reports and RN evaluations. *Intensive & Critical Care Nursing, 17*(1), 29–39.

8. Williams, C. (2005). The identification of family members' contribution to patients' care in the intensive care unit: A naturalistic inquiry. *British Association of Critical Care Nurses, Nursing in Critical Care,10*(1), 6–14.

9. Bassett, C.C. (1993). Communication with the critically ill. *Care of the Critically Ill, 9*(5), 216–219.

10. Villanueva, N. (1997). Experiences of critical care nurses caring for clients in traumatic coma or pharmacological paralysis. *Dissertation Abstracts International, 58*(08B), 4149.

11. Johnson, P., St. John, W., Moyle, W. (2006). Long-term mechanical ventilation in a critical care unit: Existing in an uneveryday world. *Journal of Advanced Nursing, 53*(5), 551–558.

12. Happ, M.B., Roesch, T.K., & Garrett, K. (2004). Electronic voice-output communication aids for temporarily nonspeaking patients in a medical intensive care unit: A feasibility study. *Heart & Lung, 33*(2), 92–101.

13. Happ, M.B. (2001). Communicating with mechanically ventilated clients: State of the science. *AACN Clinical Issues, 2*(2), 247–258.

14. Adler, D.C. (1997). *The experience and caring needs of critically ill mechanically ventilated clients.* Dissertation, University of Pennsylvania.

15. Jablonski-Seeger, R.A. (1994). The experience of being mechanically ventilated. *Qualitative Health Research,* 186–207.

16. Melles, A.M., & Zago, M.F. (2001). The magic blackboard in the promotion of written communication by tracheostomized clients. *Revista Latino-Americana de Enfermagem, 9*(1), 73–79.

17. Costello, J.M. (2000). AAC intervention in the intensive care unit: The Children's Hospital Boston model. *Augmentative and Alternative Communication, 16*(3), 137–153.

18. Kaut, K., Turcott, J.C., & Lavery, M. (1996). Passy-Muir speaking valve. *Dimensions of Critical Care Nursing, 15*(6), 298–306.

19. Passy, V., Baydur, A., Prentice, W., & Darnell-Neal, R. (1993). Passy-Muir tracheostomy speaking valve on ventilator-dependent clients. *Laryngoscope, 103,* 653–658.

20. Lohmeier, H.L., & Hoit, J.D. (2003). Ventilator-supported communication: A survey of ventilator users. *Journal of Medical Speech-Language Pathology, 11*(1), 61–73.

21. Alibali, M.W., Health, D.C., & Myers, H.J. (2001). Effects of visibility between speaker and listener on gesture production: Some gestures are meant to be seen. *Journal of Memory and Language, 44*(2), 169–188.

22. Dreger, V. (2001). Communication: An important assessment and teaching tool. *Insight, 26*(2), 57–60.

23. Hemsley, B., Sigafoos, J., Balandin, S., et al. (2001). Nursing the client with severe communication impairment. *Journal of Advanced Nursing, 35*(6), 827–835.

11

Communicating with Clients Experiencing Psychiatric Illness

Christine L. Williams, DNSc, APRN, BC

OBJECTIVES

1. To discuss the importance of communication as a therapeutic strategy for clients with severe psychiatric illnesses

2. To compare and contrast communication approaches to clients experiencing varying symptoms of severe psychiatric illness

3. To analyze barriers to therapeutic communication with clients who experience psychiatric symptoms

"Listen with compassion and an open heart, without interrupting: listening to another's story is a healing gift of self" (p. 201).[1]

■ INTRODUCTION

Nurses may care for clients with mental illness in a variety of locations, including hospital-based psychiatric units, offices, and community and urgent care settings. These clients experience the same medical illnesses, accidents, surgical procedures, and need for primary care as other clients. Individuals may exhibit symptoms of psychiatric illness during childbirth or in settings where their children receive care. Therefore, all nurses should be prepared to interact with people who have symptoms of mental illness.

There are multiple causes of psychiatric illness, including genetic influences, intrauterine and birth trauma, as well as environmental factors. Nurses use a variety of strategies to work with this population, including therapeutic milieu, group therapy, one-to-one relationships, and somatic therapies. This chapter focuses on verbal and nonverbal therapeutic techniques the nurse can use when interacting with clients who have psychiatric illnesses regardless of setting.

When clients are suffering from mental illness, successful communication can be challenging. Nurses must adapt their approach to the symptoms that clients display. Because the psychiatric client seems so different or so difficult to reach, nurses frequently experience anxiety when they begin working with this population. Caregivers' (both family and professional) emotional reactions to clients with schizophrenia have been studied extensively.[2] Caregiver hostility and absence of rapport have been significantly related to negative client outcomes such as relapse and rehospitalization. Nurses' unrealistic expectations of clients and lack of understanding of symptoms contribute to their negative attitudes and lack of caring.

Positive relationships do make a difference. In their review of recent research, Hewitt and Coffey[3] found that the quality of the relationship between patients with schizophrenia and their care provider had a significant impact on clinical outcomes. Compliance with taking medications, remaining in a therapeutic relationship, and better symptom outcomes were all associated with client-rated positive relationships. People with a serious psychiatric illness like schizophrenia want someone to talk to; someone with whom they feel comfortable and who will listen to them when they are upset.[3]

In his writings about the challenges of understanding the client with schizophrenia, Harry Stack Sullivan[4]

reminded readers that clients with psychiatric illnesses are more similar to us than we realize. He also wrote about the pain of clients' loneliness and isolation, claiming that loneliness is the only emotion that is more painful than anxiety.[4] All clients need relationships, and relationships have the potential to bolster self-worth and increase self-esteem.[5] When nurses focus on what they have in common with their clients, such as the need for love and acceptance, the need for emotional security, and the need for positive relationships with others, they are more likely to be supportive and positive in their approach.

Peplau wrote that the goal of communication is to develop a common understanding between people to develop a relationship.[6] In Peplau's view, the relationship between nurse and client was intended to be corrective. For example, when nurses help clients to clarify unclear messages, they help to correct their confused thoughts. Today, nurses focus on creating behavior change in clients.[5] Facilitating health-promoting behaviors in clients with mental illness begins with successful communication and relationship building.

Because many psychiatric illnesses share the same symptoms, this chapter is organized around psychiatric symptoms and the communication strategies appropriate for clients experiencing those symptoms. These strategies are intended to guide nurses to respond in helpful ways to clients who seem very different and are often difficult to understand.

Antipsychotic drugs that alter the biochemistry of the brain can decrease or even eliminate symptoms. Treating psychiatric symptoms with psychoactive drugs is an important component of a comprehensive approach to clients with severe psychiatric illness. Not all clients treated with antipsychotics or other psychiatric drugs will be relieved of their symptoms; therefore, other therapeutic strategies will remain an important component of their long-term care. Clients who form trusting relationships with nurses over time are more likely to take their medications consistently.[3]

■ CHARACTERISTICS OF MENTAL DISORDERS

According to the 2000 *Diagnostic and Statistical Manual of Mental Disorders,*[7] being psychotic can be defined as experiencing delusions and hallucinations when the person does not understand that these are symptoms and therefore not real. Clients with psychoses and other serious psychiatric conditions are the focus of this chapter.

One of the most common manifestations of psychosis, schizophrenia, has an impressive list of symptoms to become acquainted with before communication is likely to be successful. Lego wrote that schizophrenia presented the greatest challenge to the nurse's ability to communicate.[8] The symptoms associated with schizophrenia are also common in many other mental disorders, although some symptoms will be more dominant in one disorder than others. For example, an individual with Alzheimer's disease may experience similar symptoms to the person with schizophrenia (hallucinations, delusions, and mood symptoms). In Alzheimer's disease, paranoid delusions and visual hallucinations may be dominant, whereas in schizophrenia, auditory hallucinations and grandiose delusions are more common. In the following discussion, symptoms will be categorized as negative, positive, cognitive, and mood related.

Creating a feeling of interpersonal safety for the client is the first step in a therapeutic interaction. Many clients with psychiatric illnesses withdraw from others or are difficult to engage in a relationship. The nurse can begin by acting in ways that are nonthreatening. Sitting quietly at a distance of 10 to 12 feet communicates availability. Being available and observant without being obvious creates a presence that is nondemanding. In this atmosphere of acceptance, the client is more likely to approach you and to initiate an interaction.

Symptoms can become habitual for people experiencing severe psychiatric illness, and nurses must demonstrate patience as clients struggle to give up familiar ways of relating.[9] A gentle, supportive approach is most useful for bringing about change. An important principle is repetition. Any one strategy must be used over and over to have beneficial effects. Nurses sometimes wonder if their efforts will have any effect on client communication. Some worry about saying anything in case a poorly worded response might cause harm to the client. No one response is likely to have lasting impact. Consistency and persistence are necessary to gradually bringing about positive change.[10]

■ RELATING TO CLIENTS WITH POSITIVE SYMPTOMS

Positive symptoms are positive because they are assessment findings that would be absent if the client were healthy. The positive symptoms of psychiatric illness include abnormal findings such as hallucinations and delusions.

Hallucinations

Hallucinations are perceptions that are not based in reality.[7] Hallucinations can be understood as having some meaning beyond the literal description of the hallucinations themselves.[9] As nurses become more familiar with their clients, they may begin to understand more about the psychological issues their clients struggle with by understanding the specific meaning of a hallucination for a specific client.

According to Peplau,[11] hallucinations develop gradually in psychiatric illness, beginning when individuals call to mind thoughts of a comforting image during threatening experiences. When the stressful experience ends, individuals forget the comforting image or voice until the next stressful experience arises and the comforting image or voice is needed again. Gradually, this process becomes habitual and extends to situations in which the individual does not deliberately conjure up the comforting image or voice, but it comes to mind unexpectedly. The individual seems to be losing control. Something that brought relief during times of stress becomes a stressor in itself. As experiences of the image or voice increase and become uncontrollable, individuals distort the experience. Now the image or voice seems to be originating from outside the self. Further distortions continue, and the comforting image becomes very frightening.

From a neurobiological perspective, brain activity during hallucinations differs from normal. Transferring neural messages between different parts of the brain is thought to be impaired in schizophrenia. For the person who is hallucinating, thoughts that are expressed in words may seem to come from a source outside the person when in fact they are self-generated.[12] In light of this fragmentation in the transfer of information, it is understandable that the client who is hallucinating will insist that the "voices" are not his or her own thoughts. Arguing with the client about the source of the voices doesn't help the client to recognize reality and will only foster distrust. Accepting the client's experience as being real for them promotes a trusting nurse–client relationship. As a therapeutic relationship develops, the client can learn more about hallucinations as a symptom of illness.

For people who develop hallucinations during physical illness (e.g., while withdrawing from alcohol or other substances), the hallucinations may be fleeting and much less organized than hallucinatory experiences of clients with schizophrenia. Such hallucinations tend to be visual and are associated with delirium (see Chapter 10 for a discussion of therapeutic communication with clients experiencing delirium). Hallucinations are common during dementia, such as in the later stages of Alzheimer's disease. The verbal strategies that follow are appropriate for clients with hallucinations arising during delirium and dementia, as well as during psychiatric illness.

To begin helping clients recognize their own thoughts, nurses must avoid reinforcing hallucinations as something that originates outside of the person. When talking with your clients about their hallucinations, try stating, "Tell me about the voice you say you hear" rather than, "What is the voice saying?" This subtle difference implies that although the client's experience is real to him or her, the nurse does not share that experience. It is important to acknowledge clients' experiences, although you do not experience the same thing. For example, you could say, "You are telling me you hear a voice, but I do not hear it." With this statement, you convey acceptance of a client's experiences and contrast those experiences with your own. The goal is to encourage clients to question the reality of the symptom. When the experience is recognized as a symptom rather than external reality, client anxiety decreases.

Delusions

Delusions are abnormal, false beliefs that may be fleeting but are often stable over time.[7] Although clients' delusions are often quite bizarre, clients maintain them with conviction (e.g., "Every red car is following me."). Clients cannot be persuaded to give up false beliefs with rational explanations. Arguing or presenting evidence to the contrary serves no useful purpose and will be harmful to the therapeutic relationship. Because delusions may serve as psychological defenses,[13] directly challenging delusions may increase clients' anxiety and, thus, increases their need to maintain the delusion. The delusion can be used to help the nurse recognize a client's unmet emotional needs. For example, clients who, in reality, feel worthless may insist they are celebrities or important religious figures (grandiosity). The delusion may be an exaggeration of what clients really feel. For example, clients who feel threatened and unsafe speak of delusions of being watched, stalked, chased, or even poisoned (paranoid delusions).

A common type of delusion is the persecutory delusion. Persecutory delusions are abnormally negative beliefs about the self[13] and can be divided into "bad me" delusions (I've done something bad) and "poor me" delusions (I am a victim).[14] Persecutory delusions are found in individuals who are more likely to have an external locus of control or attribute negative events to external causes.[13] For example, a child who later develops a paranoid view of the world may attribute school failure to a personal external cause (a teacher who is vindictive) rather than to an internal personal attribute such as the student's lack of intelligence. Parents and significant others influence children's perceptions. Children may learn to be overly sensitive and suspicious or to attribute negative events to personal external causes. This style of explaining negative events becomes habitual. Still, there is much that is unknown about possible biological and genetic influences that may contribute to the development of paranoia.[13]

The nurse's communication strategies for the client with delusions should be to avoid arguments and to convey acceptance of the client as a person. It is also important to not inadvertently reinforce the abnormal thoughts by agreeing with the client about the delusion. The following exchange provides an example of therapeutic and nontherapeutic responses.

Geoffrey is a newly admitted patient in a hospital psychiatric unit. He tells the nurse that "people are following him and hiding in his room." He goes on to say . . .

Geoffrey: "There are seven people under my bed."

Nurse (nontherapeutic): "That's impossible. Seven people couldn't fit under your bed."

Nurse (nontherapeutic): "Let's go and check your room together."

Nurse (therapeutic): "Could that be possible?"

Geoffrey: "Of course it's possible."

Nurse: "You sound frightened."

In the first response the nurse takes an argumentative approach and presents evidence to contradict the abnormal thought. In the second response the nurse seems to agree with the client and reinforces the abnormal thought. In the third option, the nurse gently introduces doubt into the conversation about the client's paranoid thought. The nurse helps the client to begin to question the reality of his own delusional thoughts and become aware of his anxiety.

Case example

Mrs. Jackson, age 90, lives in a nursing home and is diagnosed with Alzheimer's disease. She tells the nurse she does not want to come to the dining room for lunch because "they are trying to poison me." The nurse notices that Mrs. Jackson becomes highly anxious when taken from her room to the noisy, crowded dining area. She demonstrates understanding by responding, "You seem very frightened, Mrs. Jackson." She asks the nursing assistant to bring Mrs. Jackson's lunch to her room to see if this might decrease her anxiety. In this situation, the nurse conveys acceptance of the person while avoiding confirmation of the delusion. Addressing the underlying anxiety helps the client feel more secure rather than challenged.

■ RELATING TO CLIENTS WITH NEGATIVE SYMPTOMS

The negative symptoms of psychiatric illness require special attention as well. Negative symptoms refer to characteristics of a healthy person that would be expected findings during a mental health assessment. Negative symptoms relate to the absence of healthy responses or behaviors and include flat affect (lack of affect), alogia (lack of speech), and avolition (lack of motivation).

Flat Affect

Clients with flat affect lack the facial expressiveness and gestures that normally communicate moment-to-moment changes in emotions.[7] A client's lack of nonverbal expressiveness can make it difficult for nurses to understand what the client is feeling. Clients with negative symptoms may avoid eye contact as well. In studies comparing the emotional experiences of individuals diagnosed with schizophrenia to individuals without a psychiatric diagnosis, both groups reported similar emotions when watching film clips. The individuals with schizophrenia did not appear to be reacting emotionally due to flat affect, but they reported similar subjective experiences.

Nurses rely on nonverbal cues to understand clients' emotions. When a client has flat affect, other means will be necessary to discover what the client is feeling. Assume that clients experience a range of emotions but are unable to express them nonverbally.[15]

Listening for themes in conversation and asking for validation are helpful in identifying client concerns and emotions. Notice words that express emotions, such as "upset," "frustrated," "excited," and so on. Ask the client to elaborate.

Alogia

Alogia, or poverty of speech, is another negative symptom.[7] Alogia includes speech in which few words are used and few ideas are expressed. Alogia can progress to mutism or complete lack of verbal expression. These symptoms can be aggravated by side effects of medication or depression. The result is a client who is unable or unwilling to communicate verbally.[16] Clients who do not communicate verbally or whose speech is very limited are easily ignored. Understanding their needs requires effort and patience.

When clients are silent, too often nurses rush to fill the silence with a question. Feeling pressured and increasingly anxious, the client remains silent. Clients can be encouraged to formulate their own thoughts by allowing them time to reflect in silence. Avoid interrupting clients' silence when you believe they are thinking and eventually they may respond independently. Informing clients that you will spend a specific brief amount of time with them (whether they are verbal or not) sets the stage for a trusting relationship. Talking to clients without expecting a response may help them to feel included and valued as a person. Share your thoughts about the "here and now." When trust develops, clients who were nonverbal may begin to interact.

Questioning can influence the amount of spontaneous communication that clients use. If nurses ask closed-ended questions (questions that can be answered with "yes" or "no" or one word), they unknowingly discourage elaboration. When clients provide a one-word answer, nurses must think of other strategies to encourage verbalization. Open-ended questions that request specific information, such as, "who?" "what?" "where?" and "when?" are more helpful. These questions foster descriptions of client experiences that can be used to examine problematic patterns of behavior.

Avoid the use of questions that begin with "how?" or "why?" These questions are so difficult to answer that a useful response from the client is unlikely. Clients may give an answer, but if the response is carefully examined, it is usually not directly related to the question. "How?" and "why?" questions require a degree of sophisticated reflection and analysis of experiences that clients with psychiatric illness cannot usually provide.

Avolition

Avolition is another negative symptom that includes lack of motivation and apathy.[7] Clients with psychiatric illnesses may seem unmotivated to participate in care or even to dress and bathe themselves. Abnormalities in neuromotor function may contribute to their lack of action.[15] Nurses need to recognize their own emotional responses to clients who seem unmotivated to care for themselves. Frustration and anger are common responses to these symptoms and must be recognized and discussed with another nurse or supervisor. When feelings of irritation go unrecognized, the nurse may unknowingly convey lack of acceptance to the client. It may be helpful to remember that these behaviors are symptoms, and when clients improve, they do participate in their own care.

Avoid confronting the client who is apathetic, but use gentle encouragement. Remember that this lack of energy is discouraging for the client as well. Provide opportunities for the client to get involved in a nonthreatening manner such as playing a game of dominoes with other clients and inviting the client to participate. Often clients refuse participation at first, but when the nurse is accepting and conveys warmth, clients may decide to participate at a later time. Providing opportunities for small successes can build a client's confidence to try more challenging activities.

■ RELATING TO CLIENTS WITH COGNITIVE IMPAIRMENT

Cognitive impairment is frequently observed in clients with psychiatric illness. Impairments include disorganized speech, vague language, and automatic knowing. Nurses must adapt their communication to clients' impaired thinking.[6]

Disorganized Speech

Disorganized speech is a prominent symptom in both schizophrenia and dementia. Clients can be highly distractible by internal (e.g., hallucinations) and external (e.g., others in the environment) stimuli, and they can exhibit short-term memory loss resulting in the inability to remember the topic or theme in a conversation.

Negative emotions such as anxiety can magnify the problem. Clients with impaired ability to use abstract thought are also more likely to have difficulty with disorganized speech.[17]

Nurses can facilitate *continuity of thought* by listening carefully for themes. Listen with your full attention. Notice the client's nonverbal communication. Listen without judging or planning your next response. Ask questions that maintain the client's focus of attention on a theme or topic.[11] When the nurse changes topics, he or she reinforces scattered thought. For example, the client begins to discuss a conflict between herself and another client. The nurse responds by asking how well she slept last night. Instead, help to maintain meaningful conversation by reminding the client of the topic. A statement such as, "You were telling me about what happened at breakfast" helps the client to continue a conversation.

Cognitive dysfunction may be very evident in the impaired language of the client with psychiatric symptoms. Impairments are more evident when the client is faced with a challenge or becomes anxious.[16] In discussions of threatening topics, clients may seem to avoid direct communication.[10] Avoidance can become a habitual way of interacting. Clients may tell nurses "I can't remember," "I don't know," or "I can't think" when they are discussing anxiety-provoking situations. To help clients communicate about their perceptions and emotions, suggest that clients tell you about the specific concrete details of a situation first. For example, the nurse states, "Tell me what happened just before you came to the hospital this morning." "Who was at home with you?" "What did you do first?" Describing specific events in sequence will help clients to remember. When they can describe the events, they can begin to talk about their conclusions about the events and what they were feeling in that situation.

Vague Language

Docherty identifies several types of communication failures that result from vague language. A *confused reference* is one example of a communication failure. When a word or phrase "could refer to one of at least two alternative referents" (p. 2113),[17] it is vague and must be clarified. An example is "The nurses and doctors in this place don't care about me. They wish I was dead." The word "they" could refer to either the "nurses" or "doctors" or both. Another type is *missing information*. A client statement is impossible to interpret accurately because the client does not supply a critical piece of information. Missing information is the problem in the following sentence: "It's the red cars that do it." The nurse can assist the client to clarify the meaning of "it" by stating "I don't understand" or by asking "The red cars do what?"

Another type of confusing communication is the use of *ambiguous words*. Ambiguous words have more than one possible meaning. "I'm afraid I'll get stoned" leaves the nurse wondering if the client is concerned about sobriety or of being physically hurt. Clients may also use the *wrong word* altogether. The client states "I plan to expire [instead of retire] at the end of the year." In this case, the nurse may have to guess what the client means ("Do you mean retire?") and ask for validation or seek clarification ("I don't know what you mean by 'expire.'").

Vague language must be clarified by the nurse to increase clear communication and mutual understanding. Each time the client uses an unclear pronoun, the nurse should ask for clarification.

> Client: "They are after me!"
>
> Nurse: "Who are they?"
>
> Client: "They are trying to kill me!"
>
> Nurse: "Who do you mean?"

The nurse may need to ask many times before getting a specific response, such as the name of a person. The goal is to have the client identify specifically who is referred to in order to clarify vague thoughts. When nurses fail to question the use of unclear messages, they reinforce this communication pattern.

Automatic Knowing

Automatic knowing is another thought pattern that is characteristic of clients with psychiatric illness.[5] This pattern involves the belief that others know what you think without any explanation. It is communicated in statements such as, "You know?" or "You know what I mean?" When clients assume that others know their thoughts, it is unhelpful because it interferes with communication. If clients continue to believe another can "know" without being told, there is no need to communicate verbally, and these beliefs may extend to other (delusional) ways that another can influence their thoughts. Clarification by the nurse is necessary each time the client implies that the nurse automatically "knows." The nurse may respond, "No, I don't know. Tell me."[10] It is important to use a supportive tone of voice and facial expressions conveying warmth and acceptance.

■ RELATING TO CLIENTS WITH MOOD SYMPTOMS

Negative moods (dysphoria) are also associated with schizophrenia and many other mental disorders. Anhedonia (lack of interest or lack of pleasure), negative self-views, and anger are all common symptoms that the nurse will encounter.[7]

Dysphoria

Clients with dysphoria often project an overall feeling of sadness or depression. The client may be able to smile on occasion or appreciate a joke, but they are depressed most of the time, day after day. The nurse may be uncomfortable with this mood and try to bring about a change with a cheerful approach. This approach is usually ineffective. The client may smile to meet the nurse's expectations rather than because he or she is genuinely more cheerful. You will be perceived as more understanding if you match the intensity of your emotions to the client's. For example, if the client is quiet and sad when approached by the nurse, the nurse can mirror this with a subdued demeanor. Offering to be available as a quiet presence or for quiet conversation is more effective than burdening the client with excessive talk. Silence can be used effectively to encourage the client to respond at his or her own pace.

Anhedonia

The inability to experience pleasure or even a complete lack of interest in activities that one used to enjoy is anhedonia.[7] The *negativity* displayed when the client has anhedonia can evoke strong reactions in nurses. As in avolition, nurses must examine their own feelings to be sure that their responses convey acceptance of the client as a person despite his or her behavior.

Avoid personalizing when clients seem to reject your efforts to help, and remember that the client's cognitive dysfunction is the likely reason for the refusal. Clients experiencing anhedonia may refuse to partici-

Carlos is a student nurse who is just beginning his clinical experience in psychiatric nursing. His patient, Jose, has a diagnosis of schizophrenia. When Carlos attempts to engage Jose in a card game, Jose seems uninterested and tells him to "go away." Carlos tells his clinical instructor that he needs another patient assignment because this patient doesn't seem to like him.

pate in activities such as taking a walk, conversations with others despite loneliness and isolation, and even activities of daily living. When an activity brings little pleasure, it is difficult to be motivated to participate. Avoid arguing or commanding the client to participate. Communicate that you are available should the client change his or her mind.

To respond constructively to negativity, nurses must avoid giving alternatives that will lead to unacceptable choices. For example, "Would you like to get out of bed?" places the nurse in a difficult position when the client answers "No." Instead, use a direct approach: "It's time to get up now." The client can still refuse but is less likely to do so. Another example is the nurse who asks, "Would you like to talk now?" A better approach would be to state, "Tell me about yourself." This directness is more likely to be rewarded with an answer, particularly if the nurse waits silently until the client answers.

Negative Self-Views

Dysphoria is accompanied by negative self-views. When the client states, "I'm no good," the nurse may rush to dispute this negative self-evaluation by saying, "That's not true. I think you are a wonderful person." This response is unlikely to have any positive effect. The self is very resistant to change and is designed to reject evaluations that are incompatible with previously held views.[9] Instead, clients must be guided in evaluating their conclusions and the methods they used to arrive at those conclusions. The process involves having clients describe one experience at a time in which they concluded something negative about themselves. As individual experiences are examined objectively, the overall negative conclusion is questioned by the client.

Anger

Irritability, hostility, and anger commonly accompany mood symptoms and can interfere with nurses' attempts

Case example

A young mother describes an experience in which she was unable to console her newborn. Kara, age 24, states that she is determined to be a better mother than her own mother was. This is her first child, and she tells the nurse that she wants to do "everything right." Each time the infant cries, Kara picks her up and tries to comfort her. When she is unsuccessful, Kara confides that she feels "like a failure." Her "all or nothing" thinking about motherhood is contributing to her feelings of sadness and defeat. Kara believes that the infant should never cry or at least that a mother should always be able to determine why her baby is crying and to soothe her infant. Kara's attitude changed when the nurse provided information about infant crying. She came to understand that she could not remove every discomfort for her infant and that different cries have different meanings. With this information, she focused on learning more about her infant's cries and trying to discriminate among them. In her encounter with the nurse, she was assisted to examine her negative self-views and question her own conclusions. As a result, her self-view improved.

to develop therapeutic relationships. When nurses approach hostile clients, they may be more concerned about their own emotional well-being and personal safety than about clients' needs. Nurses must focus on anger as a symptom rather than a personal attack. A calm, matter-of-fact approach is needed to communicate that the nurse accepts the client as a person. Nurses need to communicate that they will not avoid or isolate angry clients but will continue to work with them to understand their concerns.

■ CONCLUSION

People with mental illnesses are often isolated by stigma. Lack of social contacts and loneliness account for much of their poor quality of life. Their inability to function in social roles such as work, parenting, and even leisure activities creates a critical need for therapeutic relationship building.[18] Nurses with the communication skills to reach out to clients with mental illnesses can play a critical role in improving clients' quality of life.

REFERENCES

1. Watson, J. (2003). Love and caring: Ethics of face and hand—An invitation to return to the heart and soul of nursing and our deep humanity. *Nursing Administration Quarterly, 27*(3), 197–202.

2. Willetts, L.E., & Leff, J. (1997). Expressed emotion and schizophrenia: The efficacy of a staff training programme. *Journal of Advanced Nursing, 26*, 1125–1133.

3. Hewitt, J., & Coffey, M. (2005). Therapeutic working relationships with people with schizophrenia: Literature review. *Journal of Advanced Nursing, 52*(5), 561–570.

4. Sullivan, H.S. (1954). *The interpersonal theory of psychiatry.* New York: WW Norton & Co.

5. Peplau, H.E. (1997). Peplau's theory of interpersonal relations. *Nursing Science Quarterly, 10*(4), 162–167.

6. Peplau, H.E. (1952). *Interpersonal relations in nursing.* New York: Putnam.

7. American Psychiatric Association. (2000). *Diagnostic and statistical manual of mental disorders, test revision* (4th ed.). Washington, DC: American Psychiatric Association.

8. Lego, S. (1999). The one-to-one nurse–patient relationship. *Archives of Psychiatric Nursing, 35*(4), 4–18.

9. Reynolds, W.J. (1997). Peplau's theory in practice. *Nursing Science Quarterly, 10*(4), 168–170.

10. Gregg, D.E., Hildegard, E., & Peplau, H.E. (1997). Her contributions. *Perspectives in Psychiatric Care, 35*(3), 10–19.

11. Peplau, H.E. (1964). *Basic principles of patient counseling.* Philadelphia: Smith Kline & French Laboratories.

12. Stern, E., & Silbersweig, D.A. (1998). Neural mechanisms underlying hallucinations in schizophrenia: The role of abnormal frontal-temporal interactions. In M.F. Lenzenweger & R.H. Dworkin (Eds.), *Origins and development of schizophrenia.* Washington, DC: American Psychological Association.

13. Bentall, R.P., Corcoran, R., Howard, R., Blackwood, N., & Kinderman, P. (2001). Persecutory delusions: A review and theoretical integration. *Clinical Psychology Review, 21*(8), 1143–1192.

14. Trower, P., & Chadwick, P. (1995). Pathways to defense of the self: A theory of two types of paranoia. *Clinical Psychology: Science and Practice, 2*, 263–278.

15. Dworkin, R.H., Oster, H., Clark, S.C., & White, S.R. (1998). Affective expression and affective experience in schizophrenia. In M.F. Lenzenweger & R.H. Dworkin (Eds.), *Origins and development of schizophrenia*. Washington, DC: American Psychological Association.

16. Walker, E.F., Baum, K.M., & Diforio, D. (1998). Developmental changes in the behavioral expression of vulnerability for schizophrenia. In M.F. Lenzenweger & R.H. Dworkin (Eds.), *Origins and development of schizophrenia*. Washington, DC: American Psychological Association.

17. Docherty, N.M., Strauss, M.E., Dinzeo, T.J., & St-Hilaire, A. (2006). The cognitive origins of specific types of schizophrenic speech disturbances. *American Journal of Psychiatry, 163*(12), 2111–2118.

18. McDonald, J., & Badger, T.A. (2002). Social function in persons with schizophrenia. *Journal of Psychosocial Nursing and Mental Health Services, 40*(6), 42–50.

EXERCISES

1. Self-Assessment

Caring for clients with severe and persistent mental disorders can be anxiety provoking. Much of what students expect about clients with psychiatric disorders is based on myths or lay knowledge. Use the following exercises to help explore your beliefs about mental illness.

If you or a family member were to be diagnosed with a psychiatric or substance abuse disorder, would you tell others about the diagnosis? Why or why not?

Think of someone you know who is diagnosed with a psychiatric or substance abuse disorder. What do you think is the cause of the problem?

What do you think can be done (if anything) to help him or her?

When did you first learn about mental illness?

What did you learn from your family about mental illness?

What did you learn in elementary or high school about mental illness?

Discussion

In your self-assessment notebook, summarize what you have learned in doing this exercise. How do your earlier ideas about mental illness differ from your understanding today? How have your earlier experiences influenced your choices about working with this population?

2. Responding to Situations

A. You are a nurse in labor and delivery. A woman with a diagnosis of bipolar disorder is being admitted in active labor. The nurse manager assigns you to care for her.

What might your feelings be in this situation?

What are your expectations about how this client will manage in labor?

B. You are a home health nurse who is assigned to visit Mr. Rogers, who is diagnosed with schizophrenia. He is a 57-year-old Vietnam veteran living in an assisted living facility. Mr. Rogers has a history of frequent hospitalizations after refusing to take his antipsychotic medications.

Is there really anything you can do that will make a difference in health outcomes for Mr. Rogers?

What challenges do you expect in establishing a relationship with this client?

What rewards might there be in caring for Mr. Rogers?

Discussion

In your self-assessment notebook, summarize what you think about caring for clients with severe and persistent mental illness. What feelings can you identify that might influence your approach to such clients?

3. Practice Exercises

Write the therapeutic response to the client statements below:

Client Statements	Your Therapeutic Response
I'm no prisoner, I am St. Jude. They are following me.	
It's criminal! I won't wait till you shoot me, I'll shoot first.	
It's no use, I never do anything right.	
The voices are telling me I'm the chosen one.	
You know when the doctor will discharge me, why don't you tell me?	

12

Communicating with Laboring Women

Diane J. Angelini, EdD, CNM, FACNM, FAAN, CNAA, BC

OBJECTIVES

1. To describe the verbal dynamic between the nurse and the laboring woman

2. To discuss the vital role of nonverbal communication in the intrapartum setting

3. To appreciate the use of verbal information sharing in the laboring process

4. To understand strategic communication techniques salient to the care and procedures surrounding labor and birth

▮ INTRODUCTION

The way in which a nurse communicates with his or her patient can affect how patients respond to the care offered by the nurse. Respect and caring are both basic to the therapeutic nurse–patient relationship.[1] For the therapeutic relationship to develop and flourish, communication is key, and respect and caring are part of this communicative dialogue.[2]

▮ COMMUNICATION AND CARING

Communication could possibly be the sole most important skill that nurses bring to their profession. Caring is clearly reflected in communication skills. Selected principles of caring communication that can be useful to the intrapartum nurse in the clinical setting include:[2]

- Consider that communication is more than words; it includes language, verbal tone and volume, and other nonverbal communication modes—touch, eye contact, facial expression—that can add to the caring relationship. Nonverbal communication assists nurses in providing nursing care that is better timed and more skillfully administered.[3] Nonverbal behaviors expressed by the patient are as valuable as verbalizations.

- Show genuine interest in the patient.

- Never underestimate the power of listening.

- Explanations can be extremely useful. When patients know what to expect, apprehension and anxiety are reduced.

- Attitude can affect care and, in turn, how the woman/patient responds.

- Patient complaints are not an attack but need to be pursued to resolution.

- Good intentions can be overdone—sometimes the desire on the part of the nurse to assist a patient may interfere with the nurse's ability to hear and understand what the patient's health needs actually are.

- A shared review is often helpful—a review (with staff members) of the basic principles of courtesy, verbal and nonverbal communication, handling patient complaints, and problem solving techniques can assist with a caring attitude. Patients often rank the courtesy of the hospital staff as the primary influence on their choice of a hospital.

ASPECTS OF COMMUNICATION: LISTENING AND CULTURE

Mendenhall[4] describes techniques to maximize the listening aspects of communication. These include listening for the feelings behind what the other person is saying, paying attention to nonverbal cues (body language), attending to body language as a listener, reminding yourself that what people say is information about them and not about you, and developing an attitude of curiosity using such questions as "Are you then saying?" to act as a guide. Barriers to therapeutic communication include excessive questioning, false reassurance, change of subject, and judgmental attitude.[5]

Another critical aspect of communication is the relationship of culture to communication. All human interactions are affected by culture, and culture is acquired through communication.[6] Culture is passed on as beliefs, values, and mores by significant others such as parents, other family members, and significant others. Culture is a result of what is learned from the environment around us and how one thinks and behaves. Patients, especially laboring women, bring their culture to the therapeutic relationship, and this is transmitted as part of the communication process. During labor, cultural taboos and cultural preferences play a role, for example, drinking hot fluids instead of cold, clicking fingers and moaning during contractions, refusing medications (because culturally this is what is expected), and breastfeeding beliefs. Also, words spoken in one language may mean one thing in one culture but can take on an opposite or divergent meaning in a different culture or language.

Case example

R.M. is a 27-year-old primigravida who is from an Arabic family, and she has recently moved to the United States. She desires only female care providers at delivery because that is part of the cultural background for Arabic women. She is also concerned that more of her body be covered during the birth process because bodily exposure is a heightened cultural concern for her. She desires that only females be in the labor room as well.

Effective communication, using verbal and nonverbal techniques, can positively affect the patient's birth outcome and satisfaction with the birth experience. Communication presents a real challenge for the intra-

partum nurse. Laboring women are often in pain, are experiencing a critical developmental period in their lives, have high anxiety around the time of labor and birth, and, in general, have more stressors during the birth process. Preferences and cultural mores are reflected in the response to the birth experience. Intrapartum nurses are challenged to bring therapeutic communication skills to the labor setting.

A woman's satisfaction during the birth process depends on the type of perceived support she receives in labor and a nurse's ability to establish rapport and effectively deliver pertinent information. Nurses empower laboring women by maintaining a free flow of information about their birthing progress. The verbal and nonverbal aspects of the interaction are key.

LANGUAGE OF WORDS

The language of words in the communication dialogue surrounding the birth experience is reflected in the nurse–patient relationship. Some[7,8] have argued that the health care providers' language does not support a positive image of the woman and her role in the birth process. Phrases such as "failure to progress in labor," the term "delivery v. birth," all appear and sound degrading and dysfunctional. They imply that the woman is passive (or a hindrance) and that health care providers are in control. It is difficult to provide support and praise when the value system begins to pervade the birth language. The nurse's words surrounding birth can instill doubt and negativity or hope, safety, and control.

The power of words in obstetrics gives rise to a fuller examination of just what is being spoken to women during labor. Language provides cues as to biases and attitudes as well as issues of power and control. Additional words and phrases commonly used in labor that need reconsideration include the following: confinement, incompetent cervix, inadequate pelvis, arrest of dilatation and descent, how to "conduct" labors, "down there," and "checking you."[8]

WOMEN'S EVALUATIONS OF CARE PROVIDERS IN LABOR AND BIRTH

Mackey and Stepans[9] studied women's evaluations of their labor and delivery nurses. In this study, 61 childbirth-prepared, middle-class Caucasian, multigravidae rated their nurses favorably by 90%, and 10% were rated unfavorably. Intrapartum nurses were evaluated favorably primarily for positive participation, acceptance, information giving, encouragement, presence, and competence. Nurses' recognition of a laboring woman's need for information and the nurses' willingness to provide this were felt to be essential by women in labor. Nurses answered questions, gave information before questions were asked, informed women of laboring progress and fetal status, explained procedures, and interpreted orders for women. Most nurses encouraged confidence in the woman's ability to cope with labor and reinforced progress even when it was minimal.

The disappointments with nursing staff included nurses not respecting how women were managing their own labors, nurses not respecting them as individuals, not being present or in attendance enough, nonsupportive behavior (lacking warmth and compassion), and refusing to talk with the woman or focusing on technical aspects of care. Some patients expressed difficulty in obtaining information about their labor progress and care from their labor nurses.

Bergstrom[10] evaluated the way in which caregivers performed vaginal examinations during the second stage of labor. Providers used words such as "I am going to check you," or "I am going to touch you," and "I want to check you again with your next push." Laboring women rarely asked what "checking you" meant. Caregivers frequently used the vaginal examination as a subject of their discussion during a contraction. The caregiver often assumed the more active role in the discussion. A strategy to improve upon this common interaction in the labor setting is for caregivers to use verbal communication skills to more clearly explain intrusive procedures and negotiate with women when vaginal examinations are undertaken.

Relative to information sharing in labor and delivery, specifically second stage labor, the more that information is provided and bodily sensations are verbally explained, the more women are likely to have a positive view of their birthing experiences.[11] This information includes coaching with breathing techniques, offering advice and information on progress in labor, and verbal instructions on what is happening during labor and birth. Verbal information giving in labor centers on helping the woman feel she can handle sensations by giving positive feedback and validation using nonverbal strategies. These include demonstrating breathing techniques and positions, applying perineal pressure, recognizing realistic vs nonrealistic expectations, using verbal reinforcement as needed, using concrete, specific terms, and providing detailed information for procedures such as epidurals.

◾ NURSE–PATIENT INTERACTIONS DURING LABOR

Social interactions during the time from first to second stage labor were evaluated using videotapes in a small sample of laboring women.[12] The conclusion from this study was that the expulsive second stage of labor merits more attention on the part of the nurse. During this time in labor, communication between the laboring woman and the caregiver is critical. Listening attentively to women during this stage of labor and providing clear, verbal instructions and reinforcement aid in successful pushing techniques and better birth outcomes.

Hanson and colleagues[13] identified the theater of birth and related birthing scenes and roles to that of a real theater scene with a stage, casting, costumes, props, and a set. In reviewing casting and role assignments, the characteristics of nurses identified by women in their birth stories were that nurses were available, telling them what to expect in detail; nurses were protective, giving women the impression of competence and safety; they were informative, giving care explanations; they were trustworthy, being there to listen, encourage, and not talk down to the woman but providing support, smiling, being calm, and helping with feelings of being overwhelmed. Women in labor desire to be heard and believed. By giving positive verbal messages, especially after a long and difficult labor, nurses help to create positive memories for life. Some women remember the words and verbal reinforcement that nurses said to them for decades, and this can have a long-term impact for the woman.[14]

Verbatim recordings of nurse–patient interactions during labor were analyzed by Beaton.[15] The results showed that nurses established and maintained control over the definition of the childbirth experience. The viewpoint of the laboring woman was not often acknowledged as relevant. Thirty-three nullipara women in a large teaching hospital in Canada composed the sample population. Thirty intrapartum nurses were also part of the study. Interactions were classified according to a taxonomy of verbal response modes. A total of 9918 nurse utterances and 2183 patient utterances were coded in this study. Intercoder reliability was 95.3% for form and 92.2% for intent.

Three role dimensions evolved for nurses: "attentiveness," "acquiescence," and "presumptuousness." Attentiveness addressed the question of how well nurses and patients listened to each other during labor. There were low attentiveness values for patients and nurses. The most common patient mode of verbal expression was disclosure; for nurses it was advisement. Laboring women often revealed something about themselves such as "I can't deal with this any longer." The nurses' expressions centered on what the nurse wanted done, not reflecting on the laboring women's experiences. The nurse focused on what she, the nurse, wanted the laboring woman to do, such as breathe or bear down.

Acquiescence addressed the issue of whose viewpoint in labor predominates. The author found that both nurses and laboring women were "nonacquiescent" and directive with each other. Each interacted with the other from their own point of view and controlled the conversation related to their own perspective and reference.

Relative to presumptuousness, nurses consistently presumed knowledge of what the woman's experience was or should be. Laboring women accepted this presumed authority and knowledge on the part of the intrapartum nurse. Nurses used advisement and interpretation as key modes of verbal responses. Nurses were least presumptuous when they were engaged in comfort measures. The authors felt that during labor, intrapartum nurses and laboring patients communicated from two different and mostly nonoverlapping centers of experience.[15] Although women in labor did not let nurses intentionally dominate the interactions, patients were submissive, granting nurses higher knowledge and authority. Nurses often structured the intrapartum experience according to their own social orientation and norm of what labor should be and, therefore, controlled much of the interaction. A reexamination of interactions in labor can readjust the quality of the birth experience for women and enhance the concept of patient-centered care.

In addition, using women-centered terminology that emphasizes caring and respect promotes feelings of control and empowerment for women during labor and birth.[16] This enhances patient-centered care. For example, instead of assuming that women are passive in labor, nurses could provide them with more opportunities to take an active role and maintain control over the situation. Allowing women to speak for themselves when their care providers enter the labor room and waiting for the women to defer to the nurse if assistance or further explanation is needed would be a helpful strategy.

An evaluation of how experienced labor nurses viewed their roles was also undertaken.[17] A focus group methodology was employed. Labor and birthing units in four large Midwestern medical centers were used and 44 expert labor nurses were participants. The conclusions were that over the years, labor nurses at the expert level reported using hands-on, high touch supportive care techniques to affect birth outcomes. These nurses identified the importance of letting a woman's body guide the labor process, and they often used bodily cues to help them. Being more aware of a woman's responses and appreciating how bodily cues could affect clinical outcomes were key. Expert nurses listened on several levels, for example, "I have learned to basically look at her [patient] body language and listen." These nurses also acknowledged the power of one-to-one verbal reinforcement.

■ NONVERBAL COMMUNICATION

Nonverbal communication is often the first step to establishing rapport with a new patient. In a breakdown of messages, it is noted that 7% is verbal (words only), 38% vocal (tone, silence, inflection, sound), and 55% nonverbal.[18] The nonverbal component can be more influential than the verbal. Nonverbal communication is often not consciously motivated and can be a better indicator of meaning than actual verbal messages. Physical listening skills include body motion, vocal tone, and inflection, among others.

Within the labor and birth setting, women utilize nonverbal communication, primarily vision, touch, facial expressions, body movements, and vocal quality.[3] The intrapartum nurse, on the other hand, also uses nonverbal cues to ascertain how well the laboring woman is handling pain in labor, in managing labor progression, and the timing of comfort measures.

■ NONVERBAL MODES OF COMMUNICATION IN LABOR

Observing women's eyes during labor shows a shutting out of stimuli, a taking in of information and activity, and a giving out of information.[3] During early labor, women often take in information with their eyes. Women often reach out with their eyes, soliciting contact. The laboring nurse may respond with continuing eye contact or reassuring touch; both have the ability to bind nurse to patient.

Information is exchanged through nonverbal modes in a seeking out of information by women through eye contact. When labor symptoms are evolving, a laboring woman's eyes may reach out to verify with the nurse that the woman's bodily sensations are normal. The nurse responds verbally or nonverbally to reassure the woman and bolster patient confidence and safety.

Touch is another nonverbal mode used often in labor. Touching of the woman's abdomen during a contraction or when administering comfort measures are common occurrences. How touch is perceived in labor differs as labor progresses, especially in nonepidural patients. For example, the touch of the nurse in early labor may then be viewed as a violation of a woman's body space as labor advances during the transition phase. The nurse observes these nonverbal cues to closely monitor labor changes and progress. This change in nonverbal communication receptivity is not a rejection of the nurse, but it signals to the nurse that a change in labor is occurring.

Smiling, biting of lips, body movement, and verbal groaning and moaning all convey bodily messages in laboring women when verbal expressions seem minimal. Verbal groaning and moaning can also take on cultural expressions. Verbal and nonverbal messages are often used simultaneously, such as when a woman screams, "I need your help" and then reaches out to touch the nurse. The expressions may also seem incompatible as when a woman states, "I'm fine" but her verbal cues suggest discomfort. Verbally, one message is given, and nonverbally, another message is received.

Case example

M.R. is a 34-year-old multigravida from West Indies, Caribbean. She comes to the obstetric triage unit in active labor. The nurse notes that every time M.R. has a contraction, she starts clicking and snapping her fingers and hands along with excessive loud, rhythmic moaning throughout the contractions. This is a cultural response to labor contractions and a nonverbal expression to maintain self-control.

Concern with body boundaries, as part of body image, is a critical part of the maternal experience in labor. Rubin[19] describes the body image boundary concerns of women in labor as they relate to intrusive procedures (such as vaginal examinations), products of birth traversing body boundaries, and the contractions of labor itself. She describes body boundaries in labor as a protection or barrier against stimulation such as sudden sharp noises or touches to the skin of the abdomen. The eyes, she notes, are usually closed, and when they are open, they are often "unseeing to what is around them to shut out harsh stimuli." The contact by the nurses' hands renews the patient's awareness of body boundaries. As one example, counter-pressure by the nurse affirms body boundaries.

It is vital that both the laboring woman and the nurse read each other's nonverbal cues effectively. This can provide more specific patient centered nursing care and better targeted care measures. Nonverbal cues are part of a laboring woman's overall communication repertoire.

■ CONCLUSION

Communication between patient and nurse during labor and birth is a two-way process. The communicative pattern of the intrapartum nurse can enhance and support the caring process. If this process is less than ideal, it can limit the effectiveness of patient-focused care. Both verbal and nonverbal patterns of communication drive the process. Listening techniques, the power of culture in the communicative process, the language of words, verbal and nonverbal communication strategies, and the theater of birth are critical components of the communicative fabric surrounding labor and birth.

REFERENCES

1. Hicks, B.F. (1990). Respect: A part of caring. *Imprint, 37*, 43.

2. Flick, B., & King, P. (1998). Is caring reflected in your communication? *Mother Baby Journal, 3*, 2–5.

3. Angelini, D. (1980). In Walburga Von Raffler-Engel (Ed.), *Nonverbal behaviors: Communication between patient and nurse in aspects of nonverbal communication*. Lisse, Holland: Swetz and Zeitlinger.

4. Mendenhall, B. (1999). Listening: The best kept secret of good communication. *Mother Baby Journal, 4*, 41–43.

5. Copeland, D., & Douglas, D. (1999). Communication strategies for the intrapartum nurse. *Journal of Obstetric, Gynecologic, & Neonatal Nursing, 28*, 579–586.

6. Nance, T. (1995). Inter-cultural communication: Finding common ground. *Journal of Obstetric, Gynecologic, & Neonatal Nursing, 24*, 249–255.

7. Perry, A. (2000). With woman, with words. *Midwifery Matters, 86*, 9–10.

8. Leap, N. (1992). The power of words. *Nursing Times, 88*, 60–61.

9. Mackey, M., & Stepans, M. (1994). Women's evaluations of their labor and delivery nurses. *Journal of Obstetric, Gynecologic, & Neonatal Nursing, 23*, 413–420.

10. Bergstrom, L., Roberts, J., Skillman, L., & Seidel, J. (1992). "You'll feel me touching you, sweetie" vaginal examinations during the second stage of labor. *Birth, 19*, 10–20.

11. McKay, S., & Smith, S. (1993). "What are they talking about?" "Is something wrong?" Information-sharing during the second stage of labor. *Birth, 20*, 142–147.

12. Bergstrom, L., Seidel, J., Skillman-Hull, L., & Roberts, J. (1997). "I gotta push...please let me push!" Social interactions during the change from first to second stage labor. *Birth, 24*, 173–180.

13. Hanson, L., VandeVusse, L., & Ardo, K. (2001). The theater of birth: Scenes from women's scripts. *Journal of Perinatal Neonatal Nursing, 15*, 18–35.

14. Simkin, P. (1996). The experience of maternity in a woman's life. *Journal of Obstetric, Gynecologic, & Neonatal Nursing, 25*, 247–252.

15. Beaton, J. (1990). Dimensions of nurse and patient roles in labor. *Health Care for Women International, 11*, 393–408.

16. Hunter, L. (2006). Women give birth and pizzas are delivered: Language and Western childbirth paradigms. *Journal of Midwifery and Women's Health, 51*, 119–124.

17. James, D., Simpson, K., & Knox, G.E. (2003). How do expert labor nurses view their role? *Journal of Obstetric, Gynecologic, & Neonatal Nursing, 32*, 814–823.

18. Haber, J., McMahon, A.L., Price-Hoskins, P., & Sidelean, B.F. (1996). *Comprehensive psychiatric nursing* (5th ed.). St. Louis, MO: Mosby.

19. Rubin, R. (1984). *Maternal identity and the maternal experience.* New York: Springer Publishing Co.

EXERCISES

1. Self-Assessment

In working with women in labor, the importance attached to certain words or terms become clear. There is a lot of responsibility for the life of a mother and fetus. Use these exercises to help you in caring for women in labor.

A. What words come to mind when you picture yourself as a woman in labor?

1.	6.
2.	7.
3.	8.
4.	9.
5.	10.

What do the above words say to you about the labor situation?

B. What would you want from the nurse who is caring for you?

C. What words might upset you?

D. How would you communicate pain?

E. What would you not want to hear?

Discussion

Write a brief paragraph of what it might be like if you were in active labor. What would you like your nurse to communicate to you verbally and nonverbally?

2. Responding to Situations

Below are situations in which you might find yourself as you interact with women in pain during labor.

A. Your client, Ms. Burke, is a 15-year-old primigravida admitted through the obstetric triage/emergency room and is found to be in early labor but very uncomfortable. She is crying out in pain with strong contractions coming every three minutes.

What do you think Ms. Burke is feeling in this situation right now?

What might you feel in this situation as the nurse?

What verbal and nonverbal communication techniques can you use that would be helpful at this particular time?

B. Your client, S. Smith, is a 30-year-old Hispanic multigravida with no prenatal care who comes to the obstetric triage unit almost fully dilated and out of control. She does not desire epidural anesthesia.

What immediate words come to mind to allay her anxiety?

What nonverbal cues can you read from her, and how would you respond nonverbally?

What might you be feeling in this situation?

What cultural aspects must you consider in caring and communicating with this woman in labor?

13

Communicating at Times of Loss and Grief

Christine L. Williams, DNSc, APRN, BC

OBJECTIVES

1. To recognize common situations that result in "difficult communication"

2. To describe therapeutic communication strategies the nurse can use with a client who is experiencing loss

3. To select communication strategies that may be helpful to families in crisis

4. To critique common errors in communication by health care providers in encounters with patients and families who are grieving

Loss and grief are common in health care environments. Nurses must be prepared to care for patients during these experiences. A diagnosis of a serious illness may bring with it the realization that hopes and dreams for the future may have to be delayed or relinquished. A loved one's death or serious injury is another situation that challenges the nurse to communicate with skill and compassion. Separations, loss of freedom, chronic illness, and death are all life experiences that are accompanied by loss and grief. The topic of loss is frightening to most of us because it forces us to confront our own losses and the inevitability of the ultimate loss—death.[1]

Intense emotions accompany loss and grief and magnify the importance of everything that is said or left unsaid. Individuals who have survived intensely painful experiences can often tell you the exact words that a nurse or other health care provider said at the time of the event. The most awkward and hurtful responses can be recalled in detail many years later. Obviously, the importance of communication at such times cannot be overstated. The purpose of communication at times of loss or grief is not only to collect or to impart information but to develop a therapeutic relationship with the client and his or her family that can be helpful as they mourn their loss. Even a brief relationship can be memorable to the bereaved.

Communicating about negative emotions is difficult for nurses.[2] Although nurses are called upon to provide information and comfort to grieving patients and families, they feel unprepared for these challenging interactions.[2]

ENCOURAGING EMOTIONAL EXPRESSION

Nurses have an important role in facilitating the safe expression of negative feelings. Expression of intense emotions at times of trauma or loss can help the client to relieve distress, decrease intrusive thoughts ("repeated, unbidden thoughts about stressful experiences" [p. 191[3]]), and better understand his or her emotional experiences. Expressing distress decreases isolation and promotes intimacy, elicits helpful responses from others (e.g., validation and support) and motivates the mourner to cope more effectively.[3]

At times, it is best to accept clients' avoidance of grief. In the first hours or days after a trauma, the bereaved may experience no emotional response to the loss. It may signal a period of shock and disbelief in which the bereaved has not yet processed the loss. The nurse's role is to accept the client's nonexpression of grief. The client may be suppressing painful emotions until a time when he or she is able to grieve. Perhaps the mourner has experienced considerable anticipatory grief before the loss occurred or may fear that emotional expression would be unbearable.[3]

Another common response to loss is anger.[4] Although anger is expected, it can be destructive to relationships. Nurses can help angry clients to express their emotions constructively.

> ### Case example
> Mrs. Soren, age 92, has just died in the hospital after a prolonged illness. Her adult daughter Jackie cared for her at home for several years before her hospitalization. In the days before Mrs. Soren's death, her three other adult children arrived from out of state and visited with her until her death. Jackie has confided in you about her anger at her siblings for not being available to her mother until it was "too late." Jackie and her siblings are verbally attacking one another in the hallway as you arrive at Mrs. Soren's room. What can you say that might be appropriate?

Families such as the Sorens need help to express intense anger safely. The argument among the Soren siblings could lead to long-lasting resentments and permanent damage to their relationships with one another. The nurse's empathic listening may help to prevent expression of destructive emotions. You can explain the role of anger in the grief process to help the siblings focus on their grief rather than one another's perceived shortcomings.

Nurses can also be helpful long after a loss has occurred. Opportunities to talk about the loss diminish with the passage of time. Friends and family members have "moved on" and may expect the mourner to be "over it." The need to talk about the loss of a close family member will persist for years. For example, the opportunity to discuss a loss can arise when taking a history. The client may tell you about an unresolved loss or share a memory of a deceased family member. The nurse can facilitate healthy grieving by showing interest and asking for further details. In the following example, a nurse misses an opportunity to demonstrate compassion and to communicate about a patient's grief. As part of an assessment interview, a nurse interviews an 80-year-old woman:

> Nurse: "How many children do you have?"
>
> Patient: "My son died of cancer last year."
>
> Nurse: "Do you have any other children?"

Be prepared for guilt reactions because they are a normal part of the grief process. Family members will need to be reminded more than once that they were not at fault.

■ WHAT SHOULD I SAY?

Nurses and other health care providers often believe that speaking about death and dying will upset clients and families who are otherwise calm.[5] When nurses do discuss these topics, clients and family members may cry and express emotional pain. Nurses may conclude that they caused the client to experience emotional pain. Emmanuel and colleagues[5] interviewed 988 individuals with six months or less to live. In general, research participants said that talking about grief was perceived as helpful rather than stressful. Clients who are grieving experience emotional pain whether they talk about it openly or not. Too often grieving individuals suppress their distress to put others at ease. When the nurse introduces the topic into conversation, he or she provides clients with the opportunity to express rather than hide their pain.

When an individual cries, refrain from touching them, offering tissues, or interrupting with consoling remarks. Consoling behaviors may interfere with the client's expression of emotions. When crying ceases, comfort may be offered. Accept the feelings that arise. Comments such as "You shouldn't feel that way" or "Your husband wouldn't want you to feel that way" are judgmental and not helpful.

Crying is an important response to grief that may be misunderstood by significant others. Loved ones may worry that intense crying is a negative outcome and should be discouraged. Potentially supportive others may believe that crying means that the mourner has been needlessly reminded of their grief. The nurse can help by explaining that crying is normal and helpful.

The question of "What should I say?" is guided by theories about grief and mourning. Worden's[6] tasks of mourning can help to structure the nurse's response. Soon after loss, the task of the mourner is to "accept the reality of the loss" (p. 11). Acceptance occurs in degrees and may take days, weeks, months, or years. A family member may believe that a loved one has died on one level but resist acceptance at other levels. A nurse may be helpful by asking the mourner "What happened?" The mourner is given the opportunity to relate his or story of the loss. Each time the story is told, the mourner benefits by facing the loss and gradually progressing toward acceptance. The next task of mourning is to "experience the pain of the loss"(p. 12). Experiencing and expressing intense emotions is necessary for healing. The nurse can encourage the client to talk by asking about the loved one. "Tell me about your husband" can provide an opening for the client to cry, rage, or express guilt and remorse.

Mourners who have no prior experience with grieving may be shocked by their own reactions. Not knowing if thoughts and emotions are normal can introduce additional stress into an already difficult experience. The nurse can provide information about normal feelings following loss such as anxiety, anger, guilt, ambivalence, and depression and the importance of sharing those feelings. For the client who expresses guilt, the nurse can educate the client about normal reactions to death. "Many people have regrets after the death of a loved one. These are normal reactions."

Gradually family members must "adjust to an environment in which the deceased is missing" (p. 14). Assisting the client to think of ways to memorialize their loved one can help with this task.[7] This provides a means to include the deceased in their new life. The nurse can encourage bereaved individuals to share their progress in coming to terms with the changes in their lives. Clients may have questions such as "What should I do with his/her belongings?" Because there are no right or wrong answers to these questions, the nurse can facilitate problem-solving behavior by asking "What have you considered doing?" The nurse can help by normalizing the mourner's experiences. For example, an older adult client whose husband died asked "How can I sleep in our bed alone?" The nurse can assure the client that difficulty sleeping is a common response to loss that gradually resolves. If sleeplessness does not begin to improve, the nurse can assess the client's need for referral for additional assistance.

The final task of mourning, according to Worden,[6] is to "relocate the dead person within one's life and find ways to memorialize that person" (p. 16). The mourner need not find "closure" or "get over" a loved one who has died. Instead the nurse can assist mourners to recognize that their relationship with the deceased will be ongoing. The mourner can be encouraged to discuss how the deceased can remain a part of their life. The need to find meaning in the experience seems to be a universal need. Nurses can encourage grievers to tell their stories thereby giving them the opportunity to construct meaning from the loss-related events.[8]

■ CULTURAL INFLUENCES

Culture can be a powerful determinant of reactions to loss, readiness to receive information about loss, preference for volume of information, and attitudes about communication. In cultural groups that place less emphasis on individualism and value the collective welfare of the family or group (Hispanics and Asians), members might expect to be consulted as a group when "bad news" is related or even before information is given to a dying person.[9] Guided by the principle of respect for autonomy of the individual, health care professionals may provide information to the client alone. The client is expected to choose who to share it with. Nurses may believe it is more efficient to disseminate information to the next of kin who will relay messages to the extended family. With clients from a collective or patriarchal culture, respect for the client may include communicating with extended family members as well.[10]

Expression of grief varies widely from culture to culture. Based on their qualitative research, Rosenblatt and Wallace[11] noted that African Americans believe that immediately following the death of a loved one, family members should demonstrate their grief openly (p. 67). Later cultural messages pressure grievers to "be strong" and restrain outward expressions of grief (p. 68). For mourners of European or Anglo heritage, grief responses may reflect stoicism and emotional restraint.[12] Nurses need to be aware of cultural differences and remember that restraint does not mean that the client and family do not grieve. Be accepting of cultural differences.

Expectations about how to communicate may differ between nurses and patients. European Americans may give information directly without "small talk" whereas Hispanics may find this approach rude and cold. They expect preliminary conversation about social topics before getting into a serious conversation and the purpose of the visit.

■ HELPFUL COMMUNICATION STRATEGIES

In a qualitative study of hospice patients and cancer survivors, McGrath[1] identified themes related to communication. Participants spoke of how difficult it was to talk about dying with close friends and family. Family and friends avoided them or when they did visit, the dying person felt the need to make them comfortable or at least protect them from the pain of talking about death. The participants spoke of the need to find others with similar life experiences to confide in. An important finding was that they did not always want to talk. Spending time alone and in silence was also important for coming to terms with death. Not surprisingly, participants wanted to alternate confronting their grief with silence and rest.

McGrath's[1] participants spoke of signaling others when they were ready to discuss their grief. They introduced the topic themselves to indicate permission to discuss their situation. They avoided talking to those who seemed too uncomfortable with the topic of death and loss. Nurses can also "give permission" by introducing difficult topics and giving the client the opportunity to talk about what they are feeling. When the client introduces the topic, a nurse can indicate willingness to listen to a patient who needs to unburden painful emotions and to facilitate discussion.

Health professionals are often preoccupied with disseminating information rather than being available to listen and to encourage clients to share their thoughts and emotions.[9] Words are not the only way to communicate with the client who is experiencing loss. Listening with empathy is one of the most valuable ways to offer support.[13] By listening and observing, we learn how much information the client can tolerate at a given moment and how information is received. The nurse's attentive presence is a way to convey willingness to listen and acceptance of clients' grief reactions. Nurses convey openness to communicate by frequent checking on grieving clients and by using empathic touch.[13]

■ UNHELPFUL COMMUNICATION STRATEGIES

Any strategy that discourages clients' expressions of grief is unhelpful.[8] Talking about loss and grief is difficult because it reminds us of our own suffering. Avoidance isolates clients when they have an intense need to talk and to receive interpersonal support.[1] A client's impending death brings the nurse face to face with his or her own fears of death. Being "present" for a grieving client takes willingness to revisit one's own suffering and losses. If you find yourself avoiding these discussions because of your own past or current grief, use self-help and seek support from colleagues and professional grief counselors. Notice your anxiety in the situation and use posi-

tive coping strategies to increase your own comfort.[17] Remind yourself to relax, take deep breaths, and use positive self-talk (e.g., "I am doing a good job handling this situation."). In the following example a client indicates readiness to talk about grief, but the nurse misses the opportunity to communicate:

Case example

Mr. Jackson is a 70-year-old man who is recovering from a CVA that left him paralyzed on his right side.

Nurse (helping him to get up from a chair): "I want you to push with your good arm."

Mr. Jackson: "What's the point? It's no use. My life is over now."

Nurse: "Talking that way won't get you any stronger. I need you to try harder."

Most bereaved individuals can remember unhelpful statements made by health care professionals. Trite phrases such as "At least he didn't suffer" or "She is not in pain now" should be avoided. These statements are intended to console the survivors but in fact may inflict further pain. Survivors grieve for their own loss regardless of whether the deceased is no longer suffering. Avoid discouraging clients' expressions of grief by telling them to "be happy" that their loved one "didn't suffer," "at least it was quick," or to "be strong" for others.

A common coping mechanism used by nurses is to focus on tasks and task-oriented communication.[17] A nurse who always seems busy may be avoiding his or her discomfort with grief. Performing tasks while ignoring the person or restricting conversation to procedures and social topics clearly communicates a nurse's inability or unwillingness to share the client's grief. If possible, stop what you are doing for a moment to focus on communication.

Another unhelpful strategy nurses sometimes use is "false cheerfulness."[14] When nurses are uncomfortable with loss and grief, they may communicate nonverbally that it is not okay to express negative emotions (sadness, anger, fear). Nurses who comment "you look wonderful!" or "you need to get out and be with people" are meeting their own needs rather than their clients' needs. Grieving clients who cry during one interaction and seem cheerful shortly after may be managing their grief in small doses. The nurses can mirror the client's mood and respect their need to control the timing of their grief.

▪ GIVING BAD NEWS

Bad news can take many forms.[15] A diagnosis of cancer, the need for an unwelcome relocation, change of lifestyle, as well as loss of hope for a cure and impending death can all be interpreted as bad news. Levetown[16] cautions health care providers to give bad news in person rather than over the telephone whenever possible. Telling the truth does not mean that the whole truth needs to be told at one time. For example, after an accident family members can be told to come to the hospital because their loved one has been seriously injured and to bring a support person with them. On arrival, they need to be assigned to a consistent caregiver who will provide information. When resuscitation has been undertaken, the family members can be told that a team has worked very hard to save their loved one but that their relative has not responded. News of the death should be prefaced with a warning statement such as "I have bad news." The level of detail given to clients/families should be dosed according to their preferences and readiness.

Use verbal and nonverbal communication to convey respect and caring. The nurse should use the patient's name and address the family members by name. Even after death, the deceased should never be referred to as "the body." The nurse can sit at eye level and make eye contact. Turn off telephones and beepers to avoid interruptions. Communicate bad news in a private place with support people present (family, friend, and/or hospital clergy).

Clients and families want to be informed on an ongoing basis about the news regarding their loved one.[17]

Nurses are often called upon to explain the news that was given by physicians. Repetition is necessary because anxiety interferes with a person's ability to absorb complex information all at one time. Provide small amounts of information followed by silence. This allows the patient and/or family to absorb what is said and to formulate questions. Provide written materials or resources where they can obtain further information when they are ready.[15]

▪ CONCLUSION

Client loss and grief may be accompanied by powerful emotions. Witnessing clients' emotional outpourings may be stressful for nurses. Our stress may be exacerbated by personal loss experiences. Most nurses have been admonished never to express their own emotions when caring for clients. Showing your sadness is not a failure as long as you move beyond identification with the client's loss to effectiveness in your helping role. Regaining objectivity is necessary in order to use your experience, knowledge, and skill to assist the client through the crisis.

It is common for all health care providers to be concerned about what to say. We don't want to add to our clients' pain by saying the "wrong" thing. Two principles can be useful guides in almost any crisis situation. First, most people will need to talk to a caring listener. Allow clients and family members to talk and use active listening skills. Second, when a situation seems beyond words, the nurse can provide a silent presence.

REFERENCES

1. McGrath, P. (2004). Affirming the connection: Comparative findings on communication issues from hospice patients and hematology survivors. *Death Studies, 28,* 829–848.

2. Sheldon, L.K., Barrett, R., & Ellington, L. (2006). Difficult communication in nursing. *Journal of Nursing Scholarship, Second Quarter,* 141–147.

3. Kennedy-Moore, E., & Watson, J.C. (2001). How and when does emotional expression help? *Review of General Psychology, 5*(3), 187–212.

4. Kubler-Ross, E. (1991). *On death and dying.* New York: Macmillan.

5. Emmanuel, E., Fairclough, D.L., Wolfe, P., & Emmanuel, L.L. (2004). Talking with terminally ill patients and their caregivers about death, dying and bereavement: Is it stressful? Is it helpful? *Archives of Internal Medicine, 164,* 1999–2004.

6. Worden, J.W. (1996). *Children and grief: When a parent dies.* New York: Guilford.

7. Riley, M. (2003). Facilitating children's grief. *The Journal of School Nursing, 19*(4), 212–218.

8. Harvey, J.H. (2000). *Giving sorrow words.* Philadelphia: Taylor and Francis.

9. Oliffe, J., Hislop, T.G., & Armstrong, E. (2007). Truth telling and cultural assumptions in an era of informed consent. *Family and Community Health, 30*(1), 5–15.

10. Waites, C., Macgowan, M.J., Pennell, J., Carlton-LaNey, I., & Weil, M. (2004). Increasing the cultural responsiveness of family group conferencing. *Social Work, 49*(2), 291–300.

11. Rosenblatt, P.C., & Wallace, B.R. (2005). *African American grief.* New York: Routledge.

12. Poole, V.L., & Giger, J.N. (1999). Helping others when you are hurting: Strategies for delivering quality care while dealing with personal bereavement. *Seminars for Nurse Managers, 7*(2), 71–77.

13. Kavanaugh, K., & Moro, T. (2006). Supporting parents after stillbirth or newborn death. *American Journal of Nursing, 106*(9), 74–79.

14. Cox, B.J., & Waller, L.L. (1991). *Bridging the communication gap with the elderly: Practical strategies for caregivers.* Chicago: American Hospital Association.

15. Phipps, L.P., & Cuthill, J.D. (2002). Breaking bad news: A clinician's view of the literature. *Annals RCPSC, 35*(5), 287–293.

16. Levetown, M. (2004). Breaking bad news in the emergency department: When seconds count. *Topics in Emergency Medicine, 26*(1), 35–43.

17. Kelley, A.E. (2005). Relationships in emergency care. *Topics in Emergency Medicine, 27*(3), 192–197.

EXERCISES

1. Self-Assessment

Clients who are grieving remind us of our own losses. If we have recent or unresolved losses, we may be very uncomfortable with our clients' grief. Use the following exercises to help you to explore your feelings about loss and grief.

Has a close friend or someone in your family died? If so, how long ago did it happen? What stage of grief applies to you?

Do you or a loved one have a serious illness? If so, what losses are associated with the illness experience?

How does your experience with loss and grief affect your behavior when caring for clients?

What have you learned from your experiences that makes you a better nurse?

Is there anything that interferes with your ability to care for bereaved clients and family members?

Discussion

In your self-assessment notebook, summarize what you have learned from doing this exercise. How have your experiences with loss and grief influenced your care of clients? How have your earlier experiences influenced your choices about working with specific client populations?

2. Responding to Situations

A. You are a nurse on an oncology unit. A client is admitted who is terminally ill. You notice that you have many things in common (same age, sex, marital status). The nurse manager assigns you to care for this client.

What might your feelings be in this situation?

What are your assumptions about how this client will cope with his or her impending death?

What is the basis for your assumptions?

What communication strategies do you expect the client to need from you?

B. You are a nurse in the neonatal intensive care unit who is assigned to a neonate who is critically ill. The parents are present most of the time. They often express anger at the physician, nurses, and hospital. You recognize that their anger is associated with grief.

How would you respond to their anger?

What can you say or do to communicate your support during this difficult time?

3. Practice Exercises

Write the therapeutic response to the client statements below:

Client Statements	Your Therapeutic Response
You can't understand how I feel. I'm dying and you are not!	
I can't die. I have two small children to take care of.	
The doctors probably made a mistake. I have faith that my cancer will be cured.	
My husband is gone. What am I supposed to do now?	
I don't want my father to know that he is dying. Will you help me to keep it a secret?	

Discussion

In your self-assessment notebook, summarize what you think about caring for grieving clients and families. What feelings can you identify that might influence your approach to such clients?

14

Health Literacy and Communication

Jackie H. Jones, EdD, MSN, RN and Tamika R. Sanchez-Jones, PhD, MBA, APRN, BC

OBJECTIVES

1. To describe the impact of low health literacy on health outcomes

2. To identify verbal and nonverbal cues of low health literacy

3. To discuss various strategies for communicating with clients with low health literacy

4. To portray sensitivity in assessing for health literacy

5. To discuss the impact of low health literacy on the health care system in the United States

6. To differentiate between literacy and health literacy

Nurses communicate with diverse client populations in a variety of settings. Regardless of environment, nurses must communicate basic health information to their clients. Effective communication of health information is dependent upon the nurse's ability to tailor information to the client's level of health literacy.

What is health literacy? Health literacy is a variant of functional literacy. It has been defined as the ability to comprehend basic information about health, to use that information to make appropriate health decisions, and to find and use health services.[1,2] Health literacy may be related to general literacy or the ability to read, write, and comprehend language; however, it is important to realize that low health literacy may be present even in the absence of illiteracy.[3]

■ PREVALENCE OF LOW HEALTH LITERACY

Low health literacy is far more prevalent than commonly believed in the United States. Many researchers have found that it is a common experience for clients not to understand the health care information given to them. One study found that clients were able to recall 50% or less of the information given to them immediately after leaving the physician's office.[4] Reviewing over 100 studies, Rudd, Moeykens, and Colton[4] discovered that many clients did not understand health information they received from a health care provider. In 2003, the U.S. Department of Education[5] conducted a study to assess the literacy and health literacy of adults, ages 16 and over, in the United States. Health literacy results were reported using four literacy levels:

- Proficient, which included the ability to search through a complex document and find a definition of a medical term

- Intermediate, which included the ability to read a prescription drug label and being able to determine appropriate times to take the medication

- Basic, which included the ability to read a short, clearly written pamphlet or one-page article and being able to answer simple questions about the material contained within

- Below Basic, which included the ability to read a short set of instructions and identify what the client is allowed to drink before a medical test

The results were surprising. According to this study, 14% of the study population had below basic health literacy; 22% had basic health literacy; 53% had intermediate literacy; and 12% had proficient health literacy. These statistics indicate that almost 90 million American adults lack the ability to understand basic health information sufficient to make appropriate health decisions.[5]

Alarmingly, the demographics of this study reveal that it is the most vulnerable Americans who are more likely to have this deficiency. The groups that are overrepresented in low health literacy are older adults, minorities, the uneducated, and the poor. Table 14-1 provides representative statistics for these various groups.

People age 65 and over had the lowest average health literacy scores compared to adults in any other age category. The more educated one was, the less likely they were to have low health literacy. Income level was positively correlated with health literacy and, as household income increased, health literacy scores also increased. Minorities were also found to have higher rates of low health literacy, and individuals for whom English is their second language are at increased risk as well.[5] In the following example, low health literacy led to ineffective symptom relief:

Case example

Jasmine Williams, a 23-year-old African American, calls the pediatrician's office about her 18-month-old daughter, Brooke. Brooke has been sick with a fever all day but has not had any other symptoms. The health care provider recommends Children's Tylenol three fourths of a teaspoon every 4 hours. Jasmine brings Brooke into the office on day three, and her temperature is still elevated. When questioned about medications, Jasmine states that she has been giving Brooke "almost half a teaspoon every four hours."

■ CONSEQUENCES OF LOW HEALTH LITERACY

Low health literacy is associated with high rates of hospitalization, less frequent use of preventive services, as well

Table 14-1 Populations at Risk for Low Health Literacy

Demographic		% Basic & Below Basic
Age	65+	59%
	40–49	32%
	25–39	28%
Race/ethnicity	White	28%
	Black	58%
	Hispanic	66%
Educational attainment	Bachelor's degree	13%
	High school graduate	44%
	Less than/some high school	76%
Income level	**Poverty Threshold**	**Average Health Literacy Score**
	Below poverty threshold	205 (basic)
	126–150% of poverty threshold	224 (basic)
	Above 175% of poverty threshold	261 (intermediate)

Source: Kutner, M., Greenberg, E., Jin, Y., & Paulsen, C. (2006). *The health literacy of America's adults: Results from the 2003 National Assessment of Adult Literacy* (NCES 2006-483). U.S. Department of Education. Washington, DC: National Center for Education Statistics.

as increased morbidity and mortality.[2] The costs associated with poor health literacy in terms of health care dollars are both quantifiable and staggering. Weiss[3] estimates the cost of poor health literacy in the United States to be 50 to 73 billion dollars per year. Poor health literacy contributes significantly to the health care crisis that exists in the United States and is such an important issue that it is frequently cited as one of the national objectives for achieving a greater state of health.[1,5]

Low health literacy is also costly in terms of human lives and suffering. Generally, there is a reduced compliance with medication and medical regimens. When clients fail to understand the information given to them, they do not follow instructions, do not take medications the right way, and do not perform self-care as instructed.

Nonadherence to prescribed health regimens often results in poor health outcomes and an array of negative health consequences. Negative health consequences include failure to make knowledgeable health care decisions, decreased ability to self-manage the disease process, decreased knowledge of disease processes, greater likelihood of experiencing poor diabetic outcomes, and greater prevalence of diabetic complications, including retinopathy, nephropathy, lower extremity amputation, cerebrovascular disease, and cardiovascular disease. Additionally, poor health literacy is associated with reduced utilization of health screenings, higher rates of hospitalization, greater likelihood of emergency department visits, poorer health status, and higher morbidity and mortality.[5,6,7]

In considering the relationship between poor health literacy and client safety, Weiss[3] cites numerous studies that link medication dosing errors to low health literacy. Clients with low health literacy were unable to properly dilute a medication, unable to determine proper dosage, unable to properly use an albuterol inhaler, and made er-

Case example

Mr. Alfonso is a 50-year-old Spanish/English bilingual man who has lived in the Little Havana neighborhood of Miami, Florida for over 10 years. He was advised to take Lanoxin .125 milligram once daily. When the nurse asked him to explain how often he would take his medication, he stated that he planned to take it 11 times a day. After describing the misunderstanding to a Spanish-speaking colleague, the nurse learned that the Spanish word for 11 is spelled "once."

rors in drawing up and administering insulin. The previous example illustrates how low health literacy can lead to a serious medication error.

■ INVISIBILITY OF HEALTH LITERACY

Health literacy is not always obvious in a client's appearance, speech patterns, or behavior. In fact, poor health literacy frequently goes unreported, unacknowledged, and, therefore, unaddressed. In one study, medical residents attempted to identify poor literacy skills based on their interactions with clients. These residents failed to identify 80% of the clients who had a reading deficit.[8] Other researchers had similar conclusions when approximately 75% of those with reading deficits were not acknowledged.[9] This occurs largely because clients do not disclose the lack of understanding and may even indicate understanding where little or none exists. Many clients who have low functional health literacy deny that they have any difficulty in reading or understanding what they have read. Often, family members or significant others may be unaware of low health literacy as well. Of those clients who report this difficulty, almost 50% indicate feelings of shame, and 75% report that they never reveal limited literacy skills to their health care providers.[10]

Another reason health literacy is unaddressed is because nurses and other health care providers fail to assess clients for this deficit. When providing client education, it is easy to assume that a client understands the information provided if the client does not indicate otherwise. Misunderstandings occur when nurses are unaware that their clients do not understand the information provided. This lack of awareness results in disconnected, ineffective communication with potentially devastating implications for a client's overall health and well-being.

■ IMPROVING THE COMMUNICATION DISCONNECT

The prevalence of low health literacy could be significantly reduced with more effective communication. Nurses need to be more aware of the potential for low health literacy and adapt their communication to the client's ability level. The first step to improving communication is to assess for health literacy. Although health literacy is not something that can be visualized, there are some typical client behaviors that signal the presence of poor health literacy.[2,4,11] These include the client:

- wanting to delay or postpone reading a health-related document immediately. The client may state that he or she forgot to bring glasses or simply wants to take the material home to read it.

- taking an inordinately long time to complete documents and/or completing the forms incompletely or incorrectly.

- signing the document immediately without reading it.

- not asking any questions, even with a new diagnosis or very complicated information.

- having family members complete forms for them.

- not following through with a recommended health regimen, missing appointments often, and inability to answer questions about their medications, such as the name, purpose, or timing.

■ HOW TO ASSESS

Definitions of health literacy include the broad and complex understanding not only of the ability to read and write but also the ability to understand and use information, calculate and compute dosages, and navigate the health care system. It is important to note that health literacy is not only about one's education or how one looks. A person may be fluent in English and able to read and write and still have difficulty managing their health.

Case example

Leo Smith is a 65-year-old Caucasian recently diagnosed with Type II diabetes. He has been placed on an 1800 calorie ADA diet. Upon returning to the clinic for follow up, his blood sugar is 415. In questioning Mr. Smith, the nurse determines that he has been compliant with his diabetic medication regimen. However, when reviewing the dietary log, the nurse discovers that Mr. Smith's calorie intake has consistently been in excess of 3000 calories a day. Upon further questioning, the nurse determines that Mr. Smith is unable to calculate caloric intake or determine single serving size from nutrition labels.

Assessment of health literacy is complex because of the multiple skills needed to address health. There are three widely used tests of health literacy: Test of Func-

tional Health Literacy in Adults (TOFHLA),[12] Rapid Estimate of Adult Literacy in Medicine (REALM),[13] and the Newest Vital Sign Assessment (NVS).[14] Each instrument measures reading and interpretation skills as applied to material with health content.

The TOFHLA was developed to assess adult literacy in a health care setting (both numeracy and reading comprehension) using actual health-related materials such as prescription bottle labels and appointment slips. The REALM is a word recognition and pronunciation test where 66 health related words are read aloud and one point is given for each word read correctly. The NVS uses a nutritional label accompanied by six questions to assess health literacy. The test can be administered in 3 minutes.

■ GUIDELINES FOR COMMUNICATING WITH INTERVENTIONS/DESIGNING CLIENT-FRIENDLY MATERIALS

To improve health care outcomes for clients with low health literacy, health care personnel must communicate more effectively by providing information and teaching in ways that increase understanding and reinforce learning. Clients with low health literacy benefit from client education that is adapted to their deficits in knowledge and have even been found to demonstrate greater improvement in managing their disease process than those with adequate health literacy.[6] Table 14-2 provides a summary of the recommended guidelines.

Communicating and teaching should include the utilization of a variety of techniques and aids, including discussion, demonstration, diagrams, video, audiotaped instruction, interactive computer programs, and pictures. The nurse should engage clients in the learning experience as much as possible, encouraging their questions and active participation. Encourage the client to invite a family member or significant other to the teaching session if appropriate and desirable. Reinforce verbal information with written materials. For example, after a teaching session, provide the client with written materials.

Written materials need to be simplified. Numerous studies indicate that part of the problem is that client information (forms, brochures, medication instructions, advanced directives, informed consent, and durable power of attorney) are written at a difficulty level beyond which the client can understand.[4,11,15,18] Written materials should be written at or below the 6th grade level to

Table 14-2 Designing "Client Friendly" Materials and Teaching Experiences for Clients with Low Health Literacy

- Write materials at or below the 6th grade level
- Use font size of 12 or greater
- Keep words and paragraphs short
- Keep language simple; minimize medical jargon
- Use a variety of teaching techniques: pictures, video, audio, role play, small group discussion
- Reinforce discussions with written materials
- Prioritize information needed
- Avoid lengthy teaching sessions
- Slow down when teaching complicated or complex information
- Use a teach-back or return demonstration technique with psychomotor skills
- Assess client learning at end of the teaching experience

increase understanding.[3] Many word processing programs provide an assessment of the reading level of a document. Most commonly, the reading level is determined by the average number of syllables and words in each sentence or sentence complexity. This chapter was scanned using word processing software and determined to be at a 12th grade reading level. This material would be too difficult for someone with low health literacy to understand.

Materials need to be attractive as well as functional. Use a font size of at least 12 points to make visualization easier. Size 14 font is recommended for older adults. Paragraphs and sentences should be kept short as should the words. Prioritize the information that is needed and limit the information contained in written materials to the most relevant items. Remember that teaching is a complex process; teach the most important concepts first, and reinforce as needed.

Whether communication is verbal or written, simple or lay language should be used whenever possible.

Medical jargon should be avoided or used minimally. For example, the client may not understand the word "hyperglycemia" but may be very familiar with "high blood sugar." The educational experience should be broken into manageable pieces. Avoid lengthy teaching sessions by breaking complex or complicated information into multiple sessions. Begin teaching with simple material and advance to complex material with each session building upon previous information and learning. Repetition improves retention. Each experience should reinforce previous teaching and build on prior knowledge.

When communicating and teaching about psychomotor skills, the time interval between teaching experience and return demonstration should be short.[16] Use a teach-back or return demonstration to assess learning of psychomotor skills. An example of this would be to teach a client to self-inject insulin. After demonstrating to the client the psychomotor skill of drawing up the proper amount of insulin, identifying the possible sites of self-injection, cleaning the site, and injecting the site, the nurse should have the client verbalize and demonstrate the skill.

At the end of an educational session, it is important to ask the client if there are questions, concerns, or something that is not understood. This must be accomplished in a nonthreatening, noncondescending manner. Tone of voice is very important. Using an open and caring manner, encourage your client to ask questions. An example would be to say, "I know this information can be complicated and is new to you. It's common to have questions or concerns. I do not mind answering any questions you may have or explain any areas of concern." Also assess for nonverbal indicators of lack of understanding, such as failure to make eye contact or a complete absence of questioning. It is important to demonstrate sensitivity and compassion. The ultimate goal is to improve client health outcomes by empowering and enhancing client participation in self-care.[3]

Be prepared to repeat prior instructions and information. Understand that dealing with health care issues is usually a stressful experience; this will impede client understanding and information retention. If clients are to admit their difficulties with health literacy, they must feel comfortable.[17] Create a shame-free environment where clients can be free to share their low health literacy skills.

REFERENCES

1. Institute of Medicine. (2004). *Health literacy: A prescription to end confusion.* Washington, DC: Institute of Medicine, Board on Neuroscience and Behavioral Health, Committee on Health Literacy.

2. U.S. Department of Health and Human Services (HHS). (2000). *Healthy people 2010: Understanding and improving health.* Washington, DC: Author.

3. Weiss, B.D. (2003). *Health literacy: A manual for clinicians.* Chicago: American Medical Association Foundation and American Medical Association.

4. Rudd, R.E., Moeykens, B.A., & Colton, T.C. (2000). Health and literacy: A review of medical and public health literature. In J. Comings, B. Garner, & C. Smith (Eds.), *The annual review of adult learning and literacy, Volume 1* (pp. 158–199). The National Center for the Study of Adult Learning and Literacy. San Francisco: Jossey-Bass.

5. Kutner, M., Greenberg, E., Jin, Y., & Paulsen, C. (2006). *The health literacy of America's adults: Results from the 2003 national assessment of adult literacy.* (NCES 2006-483). U.S. Department of Education. Washington, DC: National Center for Education Statistics.

6. Kim, S., Love, F., Quistberg, D.A., & Shea, J.A. (2004). Association of health literacy with self-management behavior in patients with diabetes. *Diabetes Care, 27*(12), 2980–2982.

7. Schillinger, D., Grumbach, K., Piette, J., Wang, F., Osmond, D., Daher, C., et al. (2002). Association of health literacy with diabetes outcomes. *The Journal of the American Medical Association, 288*(4), 475–482.

8. Bass, P.F. III, Wilson, J.F., Griffith, C.H., & Barnett, D.R. (2002) Residents' ability to identify patients with poor literacy skills. *Academic Medicine, 77,* 1039–1041.

9. Landau, S.T., Tomori, C., McCarville, M.A., & Bennett, C.L. (2001). Improving rates of cervical cancer screening and pap smear follow-up for low-income women with limited health literacy. *Cancer Investigation, 19,* 316–323.

10. Parikh, N.S., Parker, R.M., Nurss, J.R., Baker, D.W., & Williams, M.V. (1996). Shame and health literacy: The unspoken connection. *Patient Education and Counseling, 27,* 33–39.

11. Schloman, B.F. (2004). Health literacy: A key ingredient for managing personal health. *Online Journal of Issues in Nursing.* Retrieved June 13, 2007, from http://nursingworld.org/ojin/infocol/info_13.htm

12. Parker, R.M., Baker, D.W., Williams, M.V., & Nurss, J.R. (1995). The test of functional health literacy in adults (TOFHLA): A new instrument in measuring patient's literacy skills. *Journal of General Internal Medicine, 10*(10), 537–542.

13. Davis, T.C., Long, S.W., & Jackson, R.H. (1993). Rapid estimate of adult literacy in medicine: A shortened screening instrument. *Family Medicine, 259*(6), 391–395.

14. Weiss, B.D., Mays, M.Z., Martz, W., Castro, K.M., DeWalt, K.A., Pignone, M.P., et al. (2005). Quick assessment of literacy in primary care: The newest vital sign. *Annals of Family Medicine, 3*(6), 514–522.

15. Hopper, K.D., TenHave, T.R., Tully, D.A., & Hall, T.E. (1998). The readability of currently used surgical/procedure consent forms in the United States. *Surgery, 123*(5), 496–503.

16. Kozier, B., Erb, G., Berman, A., & Snyder, S. (2004). *Fundamentals of nursing: Concepts, process, and practice* (7th ed.). Upper Saddle River, NJ: Pearson Prentice Hall.

17. Mika, V.S., Kelly, P.J., Price, M.A., Franquiz, M., & Villarreal, R. (2005). The ABCs of health literacy. *Family and Community Health, 28*(4), 351–357.

18. Wilson, F.L. (2000). Are patient information materials too difficult to read? *Home Healthcare Nurse, 18*(2), 107–115.

EXERCISES

Consider how you would describe the following to your clients in lay terms:

Medical Language	Lay Language
Hypoxia	
Bowel evacuant	
Cor pulmonale	
Upper GI series	
Lesion	

Develop a teaching plan for new onset diabetes for someone with low health literacy. The client must be taught the signs and symptoms of hypo/hyperglycemia, how to monitor blood glucose, how to determine insulin dosage, how to draw up insulin, and how to self-inject. Describe the communication and teaching techniques you would use.

Index

A

acceptance of loss, 132–133
acquiescence during birth experience, 126
action language, 70
active listening, 30–31
   to children, 72
   during interview, 34, 36
   self-examination exercise, 40
   times of loss and grief, 134
ADHD (attention deficit hyperactivity disorder), 74, 75
adolescents, communicating with, 71
advice, giving to children, 72
affirming the self, 35
African American culture
   communicating with families, 62–63
   expression of grief. *See also* culture
ageism, 79–80
   self-examination exercise, 88
alogia, 115
alphabet card, 107
Alzheimer's disease, 91, 112
ambiguous words, client's using, 116
anger. *See also* emotions
   with psychiatric illness, 117
   in response to information, 47
   times of loss and grief, 132
anhedonia, 117
antipsychotic drugs, 112
anxiety
   asking client about, 43
   cognitive impairment, 92–95
   cooperation and, 94
   delirium, 97
   nurse's, 21
   over client interview, 35
apathy (client), 115

aphasia, 84–85
appearance and demeanor (nurse), 35
approval of client. *See* judgmental responses
arguing, 94, 114
art, to communicate with children, 72
ASD (autism spectrum disorders), 99–100
asking questions, 41–44
   cognitively impaired persons, 115
   exercises on, 49
   mood symptoms and, 117
assessing health literacy, 142
assessment questions with older adults, 81
attention deficit hyperactivity disorder (ADHD), 74, 75
attentive communication style, 33
attentiveness during birth experience, 126
attitude. *See also* prejudice, nurse
   in adolescence, 71
   first encounter with client, 30, 33–34
   judgmental responses, 33, 34, 45–46
augmentative communication methods, 107–108
autism, 73–74, 99–100
automatic knowing, 116–117
autonomy
   client's, respect for, 18–19
   development of, in children, 5–6
   use of collective pronoun "we", 80
avolition, 115
awareness of culture. *See* cross-cultural communication
awareness of self, 11. *See also* self-examination exercises
   affirming the self, 35
   beliefs of effective helpers, 21–22
   bias and judgment. *See* prejudice, nurse
   congruence (verbal and nonverbal message), 31
   identifying with client, 19, 21
   promoting health and, 17–23

B

bad news, delivering, 46–48, 135
badges for identification, 35
barriers to communication, 45
  critically ill patients, 106
  cultural differences, 51–56
  health literacy, 139–143
  sensory deficits in older adults, 82–86
basic level (health literacy), 139
beliefs of effective helpers, 21–22
below basic level (health literacy), 139
bereavement, 131–135
bias, nurse
  ageism, 79–80
  cultural, 53, 58
  identifying with client, 19, 21
  interviewing, 34
  judgmental responses, 33, 34, 45–46
bilingual translators, 56
birth experience, language of, 124, 126.
    See also laboring women
black English (dialect), 63
blindness in older adults, 82
body movements (gesture), 55
boundaries
  during birth experience, 127
  communication barriers.
      See barriers to communication
  in family subgroups, 60
  in professional interaction, 20–21
broad opening, 42, 96

C

causal zone (distance from client), 55
cheer, false, 134
childbirth, communicating with women during, 123–127
children
  as bilingual translators, 56
  communicating with, 69–75
    nontraditional patterns, 73–75
  development of communication skills, 69–71
  early helpers, 10
  idolizing parents, 4, 5
  influence of family on self-esteem, 4–8
  intellectual and developmental disabilities, 98–100
  persecutory delusion, 114
  VOCAs (voice output communication aids), using, 108
clarification
  disorganized speech, 116–117
  as part of active listening, 30–31, 40
CLEAR communication framework, 72
cliché conversation, 20
client-friendly educational materials, 142
client home, meeting family in, 61

closed-ended questions, 42, 49
  with cognitively impaired persons, 115
  with older adults, 81
closed families, 8–10
cognitive stage of empathy development, 19
cognitively impaired persons, 91–100, 115–117.
    See also psychiatric illness, clients with
collective pronouns, 80
commonalities, establishing, 96, 112
communication. *See* therapeutic communication
communication style, 24, 33
compassion, 4
complex questions, 44, 94
concern, dismissing, 33
conductive hearing loss, 83
confidentiality, 139
confused references, 116
congruence (verbal and nonverbal message), 31
consoling behaviors at times of grief, 132
context of communication, 53–54, 72
continuity of thought, 116
control. *See* autonomy
conversational levels, 20
costs of low health literacy, 141
critically ill, mechanically ventilated clients, 105–109
cross-cultural communication, 51–56
  family communication, 61–63
crossing-over stage of empathy development, 19
crying, as response to grief, 132
cueing, 98–99
culture
  birth experience, 124
  cross-cultural communication, 51–56
  defined, 51
  health literacy, 140
  loss and grief, 133

D

darkness, adaptation to, 82
death, speaking about, 132–133
defensiveness in communication, 33, 47
delirium, 91, 97–98
delusions, 113–114
demeanor. *See* appearance and demeanor (nurse)
dementia, 91, 96–97, 113
  disorganized speech, 115–116
demographics of health literacy, 139–140
denial, 47
depression, overall feeling of (client), 117
descriptive questions, 42
despair, 7
destructive behavior, 47
developmental disabilities, 91, 98–100

difficult interactions with clients, 46–48
      times of loss and grief, 131–135
dignity, client need for, 93
diminuitives for older adults, 80
disapproval of client. *See* judgmental responses
dismissing concerns, 33
disorganized speech, 115–116
distance from client, 55
distractibility (children), 74, 75
distrust. *See* trust
dominant communication style, 33
doubt
      in children, 5–6
      voicing, 44, 50
Down syndrome, 99
drawing, to communicate with children, 72–73
dying, speaking about, 132–133
dysarthria, 86
dysfunctional families, 8–10
dysphoria, 117

E
early helpers, 10
education (client), health literacy and, 142–143
elders. *See* older adults
elderspeak, 80
emotional intelligence, 3–4
emotions, 3. *See also* nonverbal communication
      anxiety
            asking client about, 43
            cognitive impairment, 92–95
            delirium, 97
            nurse's, 21
            over client interview, 35
      asking questions about, 41, 42, 43–44
      cognitively impaired persons, 92–96
      communicating (client), 20, 31–32
      communicating (nurse), 45–46
      emotion-focused communication, 94–96, 99
      facilitating expression of, 23, 43–44, 96, 108, 131–132
      false cheerfulness, 134
      flat affect, 114–115
      isolation, 7, 79, 112
      loss and grief, 131–135
      mechanically ventilated clients, 105
      mood symptoms (psychiatric illness), 117–118
      trust. *See* trust
      upsetting information, conveying, 46–48, 135
empathy, 19–20, 88
empowerment, 72, 94
ending interviews, 36
environment. *See also* culture
      after loss (death), 133

client interviews, 35
      conversation with older adults, 81, 82, 84
      cultural context, 53–54
      establishing routines, 98–99
      family meetings, 61
      feeling of interpersonal safety, 112
      important communications, 47
Erikson's stages of development, 5–7
ethnocentric values, 53, 58
exercises (in this book). *See* self-examination exercises
expressive communication, 21. *See also* emotions; nonverbal communication
extended family, 62
eye changes in age, 82
eye contact, 55–56, 81, 98, 108
      during birth experience, 126
eyeglasses, 82, 109

F
fact, reporting in conversation, 20
false beliefs (client), 113–114
false cheerfulness, 134
false reassurance, 33, 43, 72
false self, 10–11
false statements, 45
familismo, 61–62
family, 59–63
      as client also, 29
      clients with I/DD, 99–100
      communicating emotions, 32
      communicating with children, 69. *See also* children
      as high-context environment, 53–54
      influence on self-esteem, 4–8
      loss and grief, 132, 133, 134
      meeting with, 60–61
      of older adults, 80
      of voiceless clients, 107, 109
family genograms, 14–15
favor, client asking for, 46
feelings. *See* emotions
first encounter with client, 29–37
      attitude, 33–34
      stages of, 34–36
      what information to gather, 36–37
first-person communications, 32–33
flat affect, 114–115
fluent aphasia, 84
focusing (communication), 44, 50
forced-choice questions, 42
frame of reference in client relationships, 22
frustration. *See* emotions
functional health literacy, 139–143

G

gathering information from client, 36–37
general leads, 44, 50
general questions, 42–43
generativity, development of, 7
genograms, 14–15
gestures, 55
gifts from clients, 46
glare, as problem to older adults, 82
glasses. *See* eyeglasses
grief (client), communicating and, 131–135
guilt, 6

H

hallucinations, 113
handshaking, 54–55
healing attitude in client interview, 34
health literacy, 139–143
healthy families. *See* open families
hearing aids, 84, 109
hearing impairment, 83–84, 109
helping process, 29–37
high-context cultures, 53–54
Hispanic culture
    communicating with families, 61–62
    expression of grief, 133
home (client), meeting family in, 61
"how" questions. *See* "why" questions

I

"I" messages, 32–33
I/DD (intellectual and development disabilities), 91, 98–100
ice breaker, 36
identification badges, 35
identifying with client, 19, 21
identity
    awareness of, 95. *See also* self-awareness
    development of, in children, 6–7
idolizing parents, 4, 5
illness, African American perception of, 63
imaginary friends, 73
impaired communication in children, 73–75
industry, development of, 6
inferiority, 6
information sharing, 44, 50.
    See also personal information (nurse)
    during birth experience, 125
    conveying upsetting information, 46–48, 135
    judgmental responses, 33, 34, 45–46
initiative, development of, 6
integrity, development of, 7
intellectual disabilities, 91, 98–100
intelligence, 3
    emotional, 3–4

social, 4
    communicating with children, 75
    communicating with older adults, 86
    initial brief exchange (ice breaker), 36
    silence, 44, 115
intentionality, 17
interaction skill. *See* social intelligence
intercultural communication, 51–56
intermediate level (health literacy), 139
interpersonal interaction, 19–21.
    See also therapeutic communication
    during birth experience, 125–126
    conveying upsetting information, 46–48, 135
    difficult, 46–48, 131–135
    emotional expression, 23. *See also* emotions
    family meetings, 60–61
    hearing impairment, 84
    visual impairment, 82
    voiceless clients, 106–108
interrupting, 34
interview (first encounter) with client, 29–37
    attitude, 33–34
    stages of, 34–36
    what information to gather, 36–37
intimacy
    development of, in children, 7
    levels of, in professional interaction, 20–21
    nurse self-disclosure, 45–46
    speaking distance from client, 55
intrapartum nursing. *See* laboring women
intubated clients, 105–109
invitation (in important communications), 47
isolation, 7, 79
    psychiatric illness, 112

J

jargon, as communication barrier, 45, 56, 143
journaling exercises, 14
judgment. *See also* prejudice, nurse
judgmental responses, 33, 34, 45–46

K

knowing automatically, 116–117
knowing oneself, 11. *See also* self-examination exercises
    affirming the self, 35
    beliefs of effective helpers, 21–22
    bias and judgment. *See* prejudice, nurse
    congruence (verbal and nonverbal message), 31
    identifying with client, 19, 21
    promoting health and, 17–23
knowledge (in important communications), 47.
    See also health literacy

L

laboring women, 123–127
language barriers, 45.
    See also cross-cultural communication
    impairment in older adults, 84–86
    working with bilingual translators, 56
Latino culture
    communicating with families, 61–62
    expression of grief, 133
laundry-list questions, 42
learning (client), health literacy and, 142–143
life stories, 81
lighting (environment), 82
lines, patients with delirium and, 97
listening, 18, 34–35
    active listening, 30–31
        during interview, 34, 36
        self-examination exercise, 40
    during birth experience, 124, 125–126
    to children, 72
    disorganized speech, 116
    flat affect, 115
    times of loss and grief, 134
living arrangements (client), 61
loneliness. *See* isolation
loss (client), communicating and, 131–135
low-context cultures, 53–54

M

Magic Slate, 107
maintaining conversation, 96
mechanically ventilated clients, 105–109
meeting the client, 30
memorialization of dead person, 133
memories, value of, 81
mental illness, clients with, 111–118
mental retardation, 98
methylphenidate (Ritalin), 75
missing information (vague language), 116
mistrust. *See* trust
MMSE (Mini Mental State Examination), 93
mood symptoms (psychiatric illness), 117–118
motivation (client), lack of, 115
mourning, talking about, 132–133
multiple questions, asking, 44, 94
mutism, 97

N

narrative knowing, stories as, 81
negative self-talk, 35
negative self-view, 117
negative symptoms (psychiatric illness), 114–115
negativity (client), 117
neuromuscular blocking agents (NMBAs), 106

night vision decreases, 82
NMBAs (neuromuscular blocking agents), 106
nonfluent aphasia, 84
nonverbal communication, 31, 95. *See also* emotions
    during birth experience, 123, 124, 126–127
    children, 70, 71
    cultural differences, 54–56
    disorganized speech, 116
    flat affect, 114–115
    loss and grief, 135
    mechanically ventilated clients, 108
    silence, 44, 115
nurse–patient relationships, 18.
    See also personal information (nurse)
    being objective, 19–20, 53
    during birth experience, 123, 124–126
    boundaries in
        during birth experience, 127
        communication barriers.
            See barriers to communication
        in family subgroups, 60
        in professional interaction, 20–21
    cultural differences.
        See cross-cultural communication
    identifying with client, 19, 21
    interpersonal processes of, 19–20
NVS instrument, 142

O

objectivity in care delivery
    empathy and, 19–20
    ethnocentricity and, 53
observation sharing, 44, 50.
    See also personal information (nurse)
    during birth experience, 125
    conveying upsetting information, 46–48, 135
    judgmental responses, 33, 34, 45–46
older adults, 79–86
    health literacy of, 140
    sensory deficits in, 82–86
open-ended questions, 42, 49
    with cognitively impaired persons, 115
    with older adults, 81
open families, 8, 9
opening conversation, 42, 49
opinion, nurse. *See* prejudice, nurse
orientation phase (interview), 35
orientation to reality, 44, 50, 93, 97
    hallucinations and delusions, 113–114

P

parental dysfunction, 8–10
parents, idolizing, 4, 5. *See also* family
Passy-Muir speaking valve, 108

peak communication, 20
people, beliefs about, 22
perception (in important communications), 47
permission to discuss grief, 134
persecutory delusion, 113–114
personal information (nurse)
    bias and judgment. *See* prejudice, nurse
    clients asking for, 46
    ideas and judgments, 20
    identifying with client, 19, 21
personal space, 55
personalismo, 62
pet names for older adults, 80
picture boards, 107
pitch (of spoken voice), 54
pity, 19
play as communication strategy, 70, 73
positive attitudes toward client, 21
positive self-talk, 35
positive symptoms (psychiatric illness), 112–114
poverty of speech, 115
prejudice, nurse
    ageism, 79–80
    cultural, 53, 58
    identifying with client, 19, 21
    interviewing, 34
    judgmental responses, 33, 34, 45–46
preoperative communication education, 107, 109
preparation phase (interview), 35
presbycusis, 83–84
presbyopia, 82
presence, 18
presumptiveness during birth experience, 126
privacy
    with bilingual translators, 56
    cultural differences in, 54
    in family meetings, 60
proficient level (health literacy), 139
psychiatric illness, clients with, 111–118
psychosocial theory of development, 5–7
public zone (distance from client), 55
pupil changes with age, 82
Pygmalion effect, 22

Q
questioning, 41–44
    cognitively impaired persons, 115
    exercises on, 49
    mood symptoms and, 117
quizzing, 93

R
rapport, establishing, 36
reality, presenting to client, 44, 50, 93, 97

hallucinations and delusions, 113–114
REALM instrument, 142
reassurance
    to children, 72
    false, 33, 43, 72
reflection, as part of active listening, 30, 40
refusal to talk (client), 46
relating. *See* prejudice, nurse
relationship boundaries
    during birth experience, 127
    communication barriers.
        See barriers to communication
    in family subgroups, 60
    in professional interaction, 20–21
reminiscence, 81
repeating questions, 98
reporting facts in conversation, 20
respect for client, 19
    cognitively impaired persons, 95
    cultural respect, 52–53
    loss and grief, 133, 135
    need for dignity, 93
    older adults, 79–80, 85
responding to situations (exercise), 38–39, 65.
    See also self-examination exercises
    children, 77–78
    clients with psychiatric illness, 120–121
    cognitively impaired persons, 102–103
    laboring women, 129–130
    loss and grief, 137–138
    older adults, 89
restatement
    as part of active listening, 30, 40
    summarizing important communications, 48
Ritalin, 75
role confusion, 6–7
routines, establishing, 98–99

S
sadness, overall feeling of (client), 117
safety, feeling of, 112
safety, health literacy and, 141
scenarios. *See* responding to situations
schizophrenia. *See* psychiatric illness, clients with
school-age children, communicating with, 70–71
self-awareness, 11. *See also* self-examination exercises
    affirming the self, 35
    beliefs of effective helpers, 21–22
    bias and judgment. *See* prejudice, nurse
    congruence (verbal and nonverbal message), 31
    identifying with client, 19, 21
    promoting health and, 17–23
self-disclosure, 45–46

self-esteem. *See also* shame
    appearance and demeanor, 35
    of health professional, 10–11
    influence of family on, 4–8
    negative self-view, 117
    promoting health and, 17–18
self-examination exercises, 13–14.
    See also awareness of self
    active listening, 40
    becoming a professional helper, 38–39
    children, 77–78
    cognitively impaired persons, 102–103
    communication strategies, 49–50
    communication style, 24
    culture, 58
    family communication, 64–65
    laboring women, 129–130
    loss and grief, 137–138
    older adults, 88–89
    psychiatric illness, 120–121
self, sharing, 96
self-talk, 35
senility. *See* cognitively impaired persons
seniors. *See* older adults
sensitivity, 22, 31
    working with bilingual translators, 56
sensorineural hearing loss, 83–84
sensory deficits in older adults, 82–86
setting. *See* environment
shame (in children), 5–6, 10
sharing cultural context, 53–54
sharing observations, 44, 50.
    See also personal information (nurse)
    during birth experience, 125
    conveying upsetting information, 46–48, 135
    judgmental responses, 33, 34, 45–46
sharing of self, 96
sharing upsetting information, 46–48, 135
signaling when ready to speak, 134
silence, 44, 115
simpatica, 62
social intelligence, 4
    communicating with children, 75
    communicating with older adults, 86
    initial brief exchange (ice breaker), 36
    silence, 44, 115
social zone (distance from client), 55
somatic language, 70
speaking, 18
speaking as equals, 96
specific questions, 42–43
speech impairments
    in cognitively impaired persons, 95–96, 97
    in older adults, 84–86

speed of communication with older adults, 80–81
stagnation, 7
standing close together, 55
story writing, 73
storytelling, 72, 81
    loss and grief and, 133
strategies for communication, 41–48
    during birth experience, 126–127
    children, 71–73
    clients with dementia, 95–97
    exercises on, 49–50
    loss and grief, 133–135
    older adults, 85
subject knowledge, 22
subjectivity. *See* objectivity in care delivery
summary (in important communications), 47
supervision, prior to client interview, 35
supportive messages, 43
sympathy, 19

T

Talking Mat, 85
task-focused communication, 94, 99
teaching, health literacy and, 142–143
termination phase (interview), 36
themes, identifying in client communication, 44, 50
therapeutic communication, 17–19.
    See also communication style
    barriers to, 45
        critically ill patients, 106
        cultural differences, 51–56
        health literacy, 139–143
        sensory deficits in older adults, 82–86
    communication styles, 24, 33
    context of, 53–54, 72
    cross-cultural, 51–56
    difficult interactions with clients, 46–48, 131–135
    elements of, 19–20
    environment for. *See* environment
    facilitating emotional expression, 23, 43–44
    first encounter with client, 29–37
        attitude, 33–34
        stages of, 34–36
        what information to gather, 36–37
    health literacy and, 140–143
    intimacy, levels of, 20–21
    loss and grief and, 131–135
    with specific groups
        children. *See* children
        clients with psychiatric illness, 111–118
        cognitively impaired persons, 91–100
        family, 59–63
        laboring women, 123–127
        mechanically ventilated clients, 105–109

older adults, 79–86
strategies for, 41–48
 during birth experience, 126–127
 children, 71–73
 clients with dementia, 95–97
 exercises on, 49–50
 loss and grief, 133–135
 older adults, 85
therapeutic listening. *See* active listening
thoughts, questions about, 43
time, perception of, 56
timing in client interviews, 34–35, 80–81
toddlers, communicating with, 70
TOFHLA instrument, 142
tone (of spoken voice), 54
touch. *See also* nonverbal communication
 during birth experience, 127
 cultural differences regarding, 54–55
tracheotomy, clients with, 108
transition statements, 36, 47
translators (language), 56
troubled families, characteristics of, 9
trust, 21
 in client interview, 31, 35, 36
 cognitively impaired persons, 93–94, 99–100, 115
 development of, in children, 5
 false statements, 45
 intimacy in professional relationships, 20–21
 in nurse–patient relationships, 18
tubes, patients with delirium and, 97

U
understanding oneself. *See* awareness of self
unhealthy families, 8–10
unhelpful responses, 33
upsetting information, conveying, 46–48, 135

V
vague language, 116
ventilator users, 105–109
verbal communication impairments, older adults, 84–86
verbal language, development of, 70
violence, 47
vision impairment, 82, 109
voice, 54
voice output communication aids (VOCAs), 85, 107–108
voicelessness, 105

W
"we," implying lack of autonomy, 80
"why" questions, 44, 94, 115
women in labor, 123–127
word games with children, 72
words used for birth experience, 124, 126
working phase (interview), 36
writing, to communicate, 107
 with children, 73
 with older adults, 85, 86
written materials, health literacy and, 142–143
wrong words, client's using, 116